# CALM, FOCUSED, AND PRODUCTIVE

5 Steps to Optimizing and Restoring Brain Health

©2024

## Lisa Ann de Garcia

LisaAnndeGarcia.com

**Title**: Calm, Focused, and Productive: 5 Steps for optimizing and restoring brain health
**First Edition, 2024

**ISBN**: 978-0-9860917-7-3

Published by Lisa Ann de Garcia

*Disclaimer*:
The information in this book is intended for educational purposes only and is not intended to replace the advice of your healthcare professional. The author and publisher disclaim any liability for any medical outcomes.

Cover Design by Lisa Ann de Garcia

Printed in the United States of America
**Published in 2024**

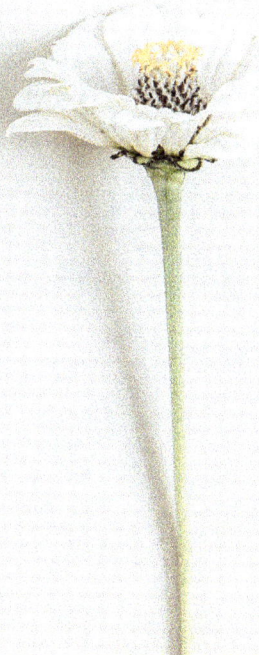

# Table of Contents

# Introduction

Welcome to 5 Steps to Balancing and Optimizing Brain Function. This book is your roadmap to reclaiming your focus, clarity, and calm in a world that's increasingly demanding on your brain. Whether you're a professional struggling with late-onset ADHD symptoms, someone who feels overwhelmed by brain fog, anxiety, and distraction, or a parent of a child who is struggling in school, this book is designed to help you and your family achieve peak mental performance.

I'm Lisa Ann de Garcia, and I've spent the last 20 years immersed in the study of brain development and health. My journey began when my son was diagnosed with autism, which sparked my relentless pursuit of knowledge in this field. I later became a learning specialist (elementary mathematics) and found that the majority of my students struggled with something much deeper than mathematics, so I started digging to uncover the world of brain development and what factors would influence learning. With a background in education and a transition into functional health practice, I've helped countless individuals optimize their brain function through a holistic, science-backed approach.

In the following chapters, I'll guide you through a comprehensive 5-step model to restore and enhance your brain health. You'll learn how to extinguish the inflammation that's causing your cognitive symptoms, detoxify your body and brain, nourish your neurons, balance your nervous system, and finally, rewire your brain for optimal performance.

This is the 30,000-foot view of what you need to optimize your brain function. While this book provides a thorough understanding, it is part of a larger framework that includes more detailed courses on each step.

Let's dive in and start your journey to a sharper, more focused, and calmer mind.

# Why Brain Health Matters

In today's fast-paced, high-stakes world, the demand on our cognitive resources has never been greater. Professionals are expected to manage increasing workloads, meet tight deadlines, and juggle multiple tasks—all while maintaining peak performance. This relentless pressure often leads to mental exhaustion, stress, and a gradual decline in cognitive function. The brain, like any other organ in our body, can only perform optimally when it's properly cared for and maintained.

However, when faced with cognitive challenges such as brain fog, anxiety, poor focus, or even symptoms of late-onset ADHD, many people simply push through, assuming it's just part of getting older or the price of a demanding career. The reality is far more complex. These symptoms are often early warning signs that the brain's health is compromised and that immediate action is needed to prevent further decline.

The brain is the control center of everything we do—our thoughts, actions, emotions, and even our physical health. When it's not functioning optimally, every aspect of our life is affected. Poor brain health can lead to decreased productivity, strained relationships, and even physical health problems as stress and anxiety take their toll on the body. This book is about reclaiming your cognitive health and empowering you to perform at your best, no matter what life throws your way.

What most people don't realize is that brain health is not static; it's dynamic and can be influenced by a variety of factors. The good news is that with the right knowledge and tools, you can not only halt cognitive decline but also enhance your brain's performance, achieving a state of clarity, focus, and calm that may have seemed out of reach.

## My Journey to Brain Health Expertise

You might be wondering how I came to develop this 5-step model for brain optimization. The truth is, my journey into brain health wasn't just a professional pursuit; it was deeply personal. Over two decades ago, my second son was diagnosed with autism, a moment that would forever change the trajectory of my life. As a mother, I was determined to find the best possible solutions for him, and that quest led me down the path of intensive research and study in the field of brain development and health.

At the time, I was already working as an educator with a strong passion for helping children overcome learning challenges. But my son's diagnosis opened my eyes to the complexities of brain function and the critical role that health, environment, and early intervention play in cognitive development. I knew that traditional approaches alone wouldn't be enough, so I began to explore alternative therapies and holistic treatments that addressed the brain from a comprehensive standpoint.

This journey transformed me from a learning specialist into a neurodevelopment expert and eventually into a functional health practitioner. I pursued every opportunity to learn more about the brain, its development, and its health. I studied under renowned experts, attended countless seminars, and read every piece of research I could get my hands on. I also worked with numerous families, helping their children overcome similar challenges to those my son and students faced.

Through this process, I realized that the principles of brain health apply not only to children with developmental challenges but also to adults—especially professionals who face cognitive issues as a result of the demands of their careers and lifestyles. The insights I gained from working with children were surprisingly effective when applied to adults experiencing brain fog, anxiety, and focus issues. This led to the creation of my 5-step model, which is a synthesis of everything I've learned over the past 20 years.

# The 5-Step Model: An Overview

Before we dive into the details of each step, let's take a birds-eye view at the 5-step model that forms the backbone of this book. This model is designed to systematically address the most common underlying issues that contribute to cognitive dysfunction. These issues include chronic inflammation, toxin accumulation, nutritional deficiencies, nervous system imbalances, and disrupted brain connectivity.

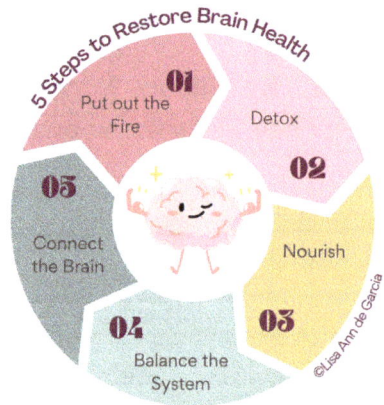

1. **Putting Out the Fire:** Neuro-inflammation is a common yet often overlooked cause of cognitive issues. Whether you're dealing with anxiety, brain fog, or poor focus, inflammation is

likely playing a key role. This step is about identifying and reducing the sources of inflammation in your brain and body, allowing your cognitive functions to recover and stabilize.

2. **Detoxification:** Once the inflammation is being addressed and more under control, the next step is to detoxify your body and brain. Over time, our bodies accumulate toxins from the environment, food, and even stress. These toxins can interfere with brain function, leading to symptoms like foggy thinking and memory problems. Detoxification is about clearing out these harmful substances to give your brain a clean slate.

3. **Nourishing the Brain:** The brain needs specific nutrients to function at its best. In this step, we'll focus on providing your brain with the essential vitamins, minerals, and other nutrients it needs to repair and grow. This step also includes strategies for improving gut health, which is crucial for brain health due to the gut-brain axis.

4. **Balancing the Nervous System:** The autonomic nervous system plays a critical role in how we respond to stress. If your nervous system is out of balance, it can lead to chronic stress, anxiety, and even physical health issues. This step will teach you how to balance your nervous system, helping you move from a state of chronic stress to one of calm and control.

5. **Rewiring the Brain:** The final step is about enhancing brain connectivity and neuroplasticity. Neuroplasticity refers to the brain's ability to reorganize itself by forming new neural connections. By engaging in specific exercises and activities, you can rewire your brain for improved focus, memory, and cognitive function.

These five steps are not isolated; they are interconnected and build upon each other. For example, detoxifying your body will also help reduce inflammation, and nourishing your brain with the right nutrients will support its ability to detoxify. By following this model, you'll be addressing the root causes of cognitive issues rather than just treating the symptoms.

## Who This Book is For

This book is for professionals who are experiencing cognitive challenges that impact their daily lives and work performance. You might be a high achiever who suddenly finds it difficult to maintain focus, or perhaps you've noticed an increase in anxiety or brain fog that's hindering your ability to think clearly and make decisions.

These issues might have crept up slowly over time, or they could have been triggered by a significant life event or change in circumstances. Either way, you're here because you recognize that something needs to change. You're tired of struggling with your cognitive health and are ready to take proactive steps to reclaim your mental clarity and performance.

This book is also for anyone who is proactive about their health and wants to ensure that they maintain optimal brain function as they age, and for parents who are trying to support their children who are struggling with learning and/or behavior.

Brain health is not something to be taken for granted; it's something that needs to be nurtured and protected. Whether you're dealing with specific cognitive challenges or simply want to stay ahead of potential issues, the strategies in this book will equip you with the tools you need to thrive.

One of the key messages of this book is that you don't have to accept cognitive decline as a normal part of aging or a consequence of a demanding career. Nor do you have to accept issues that interfere with your or your child's learning. With the right approach, you can not only halt the progression of these issues but also reverse them, achieving a state of brain health that you may not have experienced in years.

## What You'll Gain From This Book

By the end of this book, you'll have a deep understanding of the factors that contribute to brain health and how to address them in a systematic way. You'll learn how to identify the sources of inflammation in your life and reduce their impact, how to detoxify your body and brain from harmful substances, and how to nourish your brain with the nutrients it needs to function at its best.

You'll also discover how to balance your nervous system, reducing the effects of chronic stress on your mind and body. And finally, you'll learn techniques for enhancing brain connectivity and neuroplasticity, allowing you to improve your focus, memory, and overall cognitive function.

But perhaps most importantly, you'll gain confidence in your ability to take control of your brain health. You'll no longer feel at the mercy of brain fog, anxiety, or poor focus. Instead, you'll have a clear, actionable plan that you can follow to achieve lasting brain health and function.

## How to Use This Book

This book is designed to be both informative and practical. Each chapter provides not only the theory behind brain optimization but also actionable steps that you can start implementing right away. I recommend reading the book from start to finish to get a comprehensive understanding of the 5-step model, but feel free to jump to specific chapters if you're dealing with a particular issue.

At the end of each chapter, you'll find exercises, tips, and resources to help you apply what you've learned. These are designed to be simple yet effective, allowing you to integrate brain-healthy habits into your daily routine without feeling overwhelmed.

Throughout the book, you'll also find case studies and examples of individuals who have successfully implemented these strategies and seen significant improvements in their cognitive function. These stories are meant to inspire and motivate you, showing you that it is possible to overcome cognitive challenges and achieve a state of optimal brain health.

## Final Thoughts Before We Begin

I'm incredibly excited to share this journey with you. Optimizing your brain function is one of the most empowering things you can do for yourself. It not only improves your work performance but also enhances every aspect of your life, from your relationships to your personal sense of well-being.

As you read through this book and start implementing the strategies I share, remember that brain health is a journey. It takes time, commitment, and a willingness to experiment with what works best for you. But the rewards—greater clarity, focus, calm, and cognitive sharpness—are well worth the effort.

Let's get started on this journey to a healthier, more optimized brain. Your future self will thank you.

# 1

# The Iceberg Model of Brain Health and Development

## Understanding the Iceberg Model

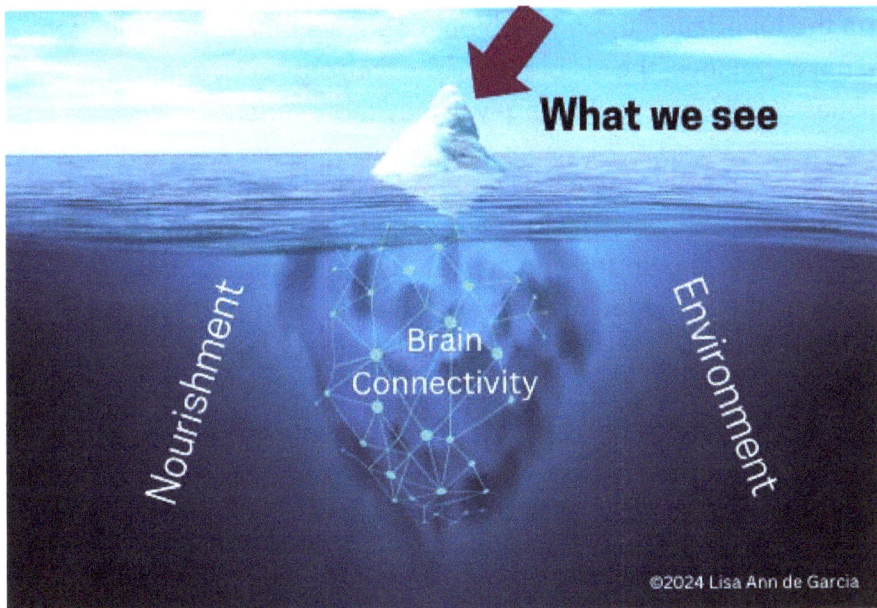

When it comes to brain health, it's easy to focus solely on the symptoms we experience—things like brain fog, anxiety, and poor focus. However, much like an iceberg, where the majority of its mass lies hidden beneath the surface, the true causes of brain health issues are often not immediately visible. Understanding this "iceberg model" of brain health is crucial for addressing the root causes of cognitive dysfunction and optimizing brain performance.

The iceberg model is a metaphor for the layers of influence on our brain health. The visible part of the iceberg represents the symptoms and behaviors that we can observe: our mood, cognitive abilities, productivity, and overall mental performance. These are the aspects of brain health that most people notice and try to manage directly.

Beneath the surface lies a complex network of factors that profoundly influence brain health but are often overlooked. These include our nutrition, environmental exposures, lifestyle choices, stress levels, sleep quality, and genetic predispositions. Together, these factors form the foundation upon which our cognitive function is built. If they are not in balance, the visible tip of the iceberg–our cognitive abilities and mental well-being–will inevitably suffer.

The iceberg model teaches us that addressing brain health requires a holistic approach, one that looks beyond the surface symptoms and digs deep into the underlying causes. By understanding and managing these hidden factors, we can create a strong foundation for lasting cognitive health and optimal brain performance.

# The Tip of the Iceberg: Symptoms of Cognitive Dysfunction

Let's start by examining the tip of the iceberg–the symptoms of cognitive dysfunction that you might be experiencing. These symptoms are often the first indication that something is amiss with your brain health. Common symptoms include:

- **Brain Fog:** One of the most common complaints among professionals, and those over 40, is brain fog, which is characterized by a lack of mental clarity, forgetfulness, and an inability to focus. It's like trying to think through a thick mist where everything feels slow and difficult. Brain fog can be particularly frustrating because it affects your ability to think clearly, make decisions, and be productive.

- **Anxiety:** Anxiety is a rapidly increasing symptom among all age groups. This can manifest as a constant sense of worry, fear, or unease, which can interfere with your ability to focus and perform at your best. Anxiety often comes with physical symptoms as well, such as increased heart rate, sweating, and difficulty sleeping, which can further exacerbate cognitive issues.
- **Poor Focus and Attention:** Struggling to concentrate on tasks, getting easily distracted, or finding it hard to stay on track are signs that your brain's focus mechanisms are not functioning optimally. This can lead to decreased productivity and frustration as you struggle to complete tasks that once felt manageable.
- **Memory Problems:** Memory issues, such as forgetting names, appointments, or even important work tasks, can be particularly concerning. These lapses in memory may be subtle at first but can become more frequent and disruptive over time, indicating underlying issues with brain health.
- **Mood Swings:** Fluctuations in mood, such as irritability, depression, or sudden outbursts of anger, can also indicate underlying issues with brain health. These mood swings can affect your relationships, your work environment, and your overall quality of life.
- **Physical Symptoms:** Cognitive dysfunction can also manifest in physical symptoms, such as headaches, fatigue, or even gastrointestinal issues. The brain and body are deeply interconnected, and when one is out of balance, the other often follows suit.

These symptoms, while concerning, are just the visible part of a much larger issue. They are the signals that your brain is sending, telling you that something needs to be addressed at a deeper level. However, many people try to manage these symptoms directly, using quick fixes like caffeine, over-the-counter medications, or even prescription drugs. While these solutions may provide temporary relief, they do not address the root causes of cognitive dysfunction and often lead to a cycle of dependency and worsening symptoms over time.

# Beneath the Surface: The Hidden Influencers of Brain Health

To truly understand brain health, we must look beneath the surface at the hidden influencers that shape our cognitive function. These underlying factors are often interconnected and can have a profound impact on how our brains function on a daily basis. Let's explore these hidden influencers in more detail:

### 1. Nutritional Status

**Dietary Deficiencies:** The brain requires a steady supply of nutrients to function properly. Essential vitamins and minerals like B vitamins, magnesium, zinc, and omega-3 fatty acids play critical roles in cognitive function. For example, omega-3 fatty acids, particularly DHA, are essential for maintaining the structure and function of brain cells. B vitamins are involved in neurotransmitter production and energy metabolism, while magnesium helps regulate neurotransmitters and supports healthy brain function. When your diet lacks these nutrients, your brain's performance can suffer. Over time, even slight deficiencies can lead to significant cognitive issues.

**Blood Sugar Regulation:** The brain is highly sensitive to fluctuations in blood sugar levels. Poor dietary habits, such as consuming too many refined carbohydrates and sugars, can lead to spikes and crashes in blood sugar, which can impair cognitive function and mood stability. Maintaining stable blood sugar levels is crucial for brain health, as the brain relies on a constant supply of glucose for energy. When blood sugar levels drop too low, the brain's ability to function optimally is compromised, leading to symptoms like brain fog, irritability, and fatigue.

## 2. Environmental Exposures

**Toxins and Chemicals:** Exposure to environmental toxins, such as heavy metals, pesticides, and air pollutants, can have a detrimental effect on brain health. These toxins can accumulate in the brain and disrupt neural function, leading to symptoms like brain fog and anxiety. For example, exposure to mercury and lead has been linked to cognitive decline, while pesticides and other chemicals can interfere with the body's hormonal balance, which in turn affects brain function.

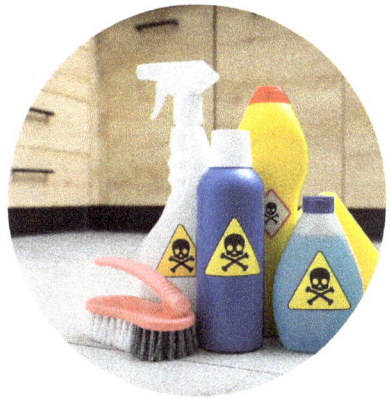

**Electromagnetic Fields (EMFs):** Prolonged exposure to EMFs from devices like smartphones, Wi-Fi, and computers is a growing concern for brain health. EMFs can alter brain wave patterns and contribute to cognitive dysfunction. Research has shown that EMF exposure can lead to changes in brain activity, sleep disturbances, and even increased oxidative stress, which can damage brain cells. EMF is also known to affect the calcium ion channels of the cell wall and negatively affect our DNA. While the full extent of EMF exposure on brain health is still being studied, it's clear that minimizing exposure is a prudent step for maintaining cognitive health.

## 3. Lifestyle Factors

**Stress:** Chronic stress is one of the most significant contributors to cognitive decline. Stress triggers the release of cortisol, a hormone that, in high levels over time, can damage brain cells and impair cognitive function. Cortisol is particularly harmful to the hippocampus, the part of the brain responsible for memory and learning. Prolonged stress can lead to a shrinking of the hippocampus, resulting in memory problems and difficulty concentrating. Additionally, chronic stress can disrupt sleep, increase inflammation, and lead to unhealthy coping mechanisms, such as poor diet and lack of exercise, all of which further harm brain health.

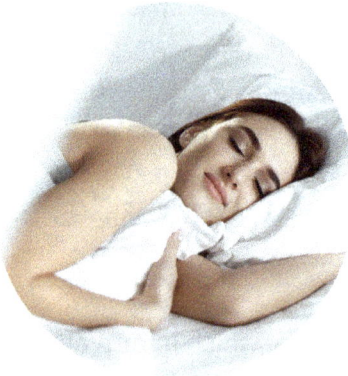

**Sleep Quality:** The brain relies on sleep to repair itself, consolidate memories, and clear out toxins. During sleep, the brain goes through various stages that are essential for different aspects of cognitive function. For example, deep sleep is crucial for physical repair and growth, while REM sleep is important for memory consolidation and emotional processing. Poor sleep quality or insufficient sleep can lead to decreased cognitive performance, increased anxiety, and even long-term health problems like heart disease and diabetes. Addressing sleep issues is a critical component of any brain health strategy.

**Physical Activity:** Regular exercise is essential for brain health. It promotes blood flow to the brain, supports neurogenesis (the creation of new neurons), and reduces inflammation. Exercise also stimulates the release of BDNF, "miracle-grow" for the brain, endorphins and other neurotransmitters that enhance mood and cognitive function. A sedentary lifestyle, on the other hand, can lead to a decline in cognitive function, as well as increased risk of conditions like obesity, diabetes, and cardiovascular disease, all of which negatively impact brain health. Incorporating regular physical activity into your routine is one of the most effective ways to support brain health and overall well-being.

## 4. Psychological and Emotional Health

**Trauma and Chronic Stress:** Past trauma or ongoing stress can have long-lasting effects on brain health. These experiences can alter brain structures, such as the hippocampus and amygdala, which are involved in memory and emotional regulation. Trauma can lead to changes in the brain's wiring, resulting in heightened stress responses, anxiety, and difficulty processing emotions. Over time, these changes can contribute to cognitive decline and increase the risk of mental health disorders, such as depression and PTSD. Addressing unresolved trauma and managing stress through therapy, mindfulness, and other techniques is crucial for maintaining cognitive health.

**Social Connections:** Human brains are wired for social interaction. Loneliness and social isolation can negatively impact cognitive function and increase the risk of mental health issues like depression and anxiety. Social connections provide emotional support, reduce stress, and stimulate cognitive function through conversation and shared activities. Engaging in meaningful social interactions can help keep

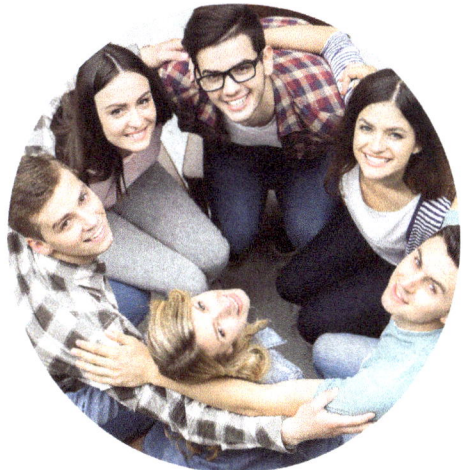

the brain active and resilient, while also providing a sense of purpose and belonging.

## 5. Biological and Genetic Factors

**Hormonal Imbalances:** Hormones play a crucial role in brain function. Imbalances in hormones like thyroid hormones, sex hormones (estrogen, testosterone), and adrenal hormones can lead to cognitive issues. For example, low thyroid function (hypothyroidism) is associated with symptoms like brain fog, depression, and memory problems. Similarly, fluctuations in estrogen levels during menopause can affect mood, memory, and concentration. Addressing hormonal imbalances through medical treatment, lifestyle changes, and targeted supplements can help restore cognitive function and improve overall well-being.

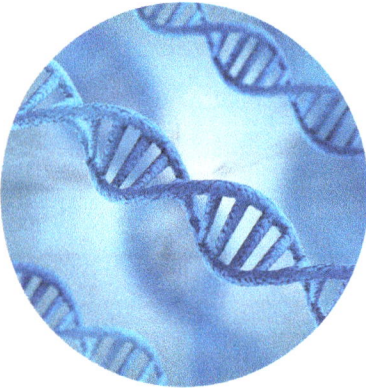

**Genetic Predispositions:** While lifestyle factors play a significant role, genetic predispositions can also influence brain health. For example, certain genetic variations can make individuals more susceptible to conditions like ADHD, depression, or Alzheimer's disease. Understanding your genetic risks can help you take proactive steps to mitigate these risks through targeted lifestyle changes, such as optimizing your diet, managing stress, and staying mentally active. Genetic testing and counseling can also provide valuable insights into how your unique genetic makeup affects your brain health and guide personalized interventions. It is said that "genetics load the gun, but lifestyle pulls the trigger."

These underlying factors are deeply interconnected, and addressing them requires a comprehensive, multi-faceted approach. By focusing on the root causes of cognitive dysfunction, rather than just the symptoms, you can create a solid foundation for long-term brain health and cognitive resilience.

## The Dynamic Nature of Brain Health

One of the most important concepts to understand about brain health is its dynamic nature. Brain health is not static; it's constantly changing based on the inputs it receives. These inputs can either support or hinder its function. For example, a nutrient-rich diet, regular exercise, and quality sleep can enhance brain health, while chronic stress, poor nutrition, and toxin exposure can impair it.

The brain's adaptability is known as neuroplasticity—the ability to reorganize itself by forming new neural connections. This means that even if you've experienced cognitive decline or dysfunction, there's always potential for improvement. By making positive changes to your lifestyle, environment, and diet, you can support your brain's ability to heal and function optimally.

## Case Study: Amber's Journey to Cognitive Clarity

To illustrate how the iceberg model works in practice, let's look at the story of Amber, a 42-year-old marketing executive who was struggling with brain fog, anxiety, and poor focus. She had always been a high achiever, but over the past few years, noticed a decline in her cognitive abilities. She found it increasingly difficult to concentrate at work, her memory was slipping, and she often felt overwhelmed by anxiety.

Amber's symptoms were affecting her performance at work and her relationships at home. She tried various strategies to cope, including drinking more coffee to stay alert and using meditation apps to manage her anxiety, but nothing seemed to work long-term. Frustrated, she decided to seek help and began working with a functional health practitioner who helped her identify hidden stressors that were impacting both her physical and mental wellbeing.

Through a comprehensive assessment, they discovered several underlying factors contributing to Amber's symptoms:

**Nutritional Deficiencies:** Amber's diet was lacking in key nutrients essential for brain health, particularly omega-3 fatty acids and B vitamins. Her practitioner recommended dietary changes, including adding more fatty fish, leafy greens, and nuts to her diet, along with targeted supplements to address these deficiencies.

**High Stress Levels:** Amber's job was extremely demanding, and she had been operating in a state of chronic stress for years, which was taking a toll on her brain. Her practitioner worked with her to develop a stress management plan that included mindfulness meditation, breathing exercises, and regular breaks during the workday to reduce her cortisol levels.

**Poor Sleep:** Amber was getting less than six hours of sleep per night, and her sleep quality was poor due to late-night screen use. She was advised to establish a regular sleep schedule, reduce screen time before bed, and create a relaxing bedtime routine to improve her sleep quality.

**Toxin Exposure:** Amber lived in a busy city and was exposed to air pollution and other environmental toxins on a daily basis. To address this, she started using an air purifier in her home, switched to natural cleaning products, and took steps to reduce her overall exposure to environmental toxins.

**Sedentary Lifestyle:** Due to her busy schedule, Amber rarely found time for exercise, contributing to her cognitive decline. Her practitioner encouraged her to incorporate regular physical activity into her routine, starting with short walks during her lunch break and gradually increasing her exercise intensity over time.

Working with her practitioner, Amber implemented a plan to address these underlying issues. She started by adjusting her diet to include more brain-healthy foods, started a supplement protocol to help provide the nutrients needed for repair,  began a regular exercise routine, and made changes to improve her sleep hygiene. She also started using stress management techniques, such as mindfulness and deep breathing exercises, to lower her cortisol levels.

Over the next few months, Amber noticed a significant improvement in her cognitive function. Her brain fog lifted, her focus improved, and her anxiety decreased. By addressing the factors beneath the surface of the iceberg, Amber was able to transform her brain health and reclaim her cognitive clarity.

# The Power of a Comprehensive Approach

The iceberg model teaches us that brain health is complex and multifaceted. It's not just about addressing the symptoms that are visible above the surface but about understanding and managing the underlying factors that contribute to those symptoms. By taking a comprehensive approach to brain health, you can make lasting changes that go beyond temporary fixes and lead to long-term cognitive resilience and well-being.

This approach requires patience and commitment, as it involves making changes to multiple aspects of your life. However, the benefits of addressing the underlying causes of cognitive dysfunction are profound. Not only can you improve your cognitive performance, but you can also enhance your overall quality of life, reduce your risk of chronic diseases, and achieve a greater sense of mental and emotional well-being.

In the following chapters, we'll delve deeper into the 5-step model for balancing and optimizing brain function. Each step builds on the understanding of the iceberg model, guiding you through a systematic approach to transform your brain health from the inside out. By addressing each layer of the iceberg, you can create a solid foundation for a healthier, more resilient brain that supports you in all aspects of your life.

# 2

## Step 1
## – Putting Out the Fire

### Introduction to Neuro-Inflammation

Imagine your brain is like a bustling city. It's full of energy, activity, and interconnected systems all working together to keep everything running smoothly. Now, imagine that a fire starts in one of the city's key areas. At first, it might be small—just a few flames—but if left unchecked, it can spread rapidly, causing damage to structures, disrupting traffic, and ultimately bringing the entire city to a standstill.

This is what happens when neuro-inflammation takes hold in the brain. Neuro-inflammation is essentially your brain's response to various types of damage or threats. While inflammation is a natural part of the body's immune response, designed to protect and heal, chronic inflammation in the brain is like that fire—it can cause widespread disruption, leading to symptoms like anxiety, brain fog, poor focus, and more.

It is important to note that if there is inflammation happening in the brain, it most likely is not an isolated event, rather inflammation is happening systemically.  So it is important to consider the entire body when it comes to dealing with inflammation.

Understanding and managing neuro-inflammation is the first and most critical step in restoring and optimizing brain function. This chapter will explore the causes of neuro-inflammation, its impact on cognitive health, and practical strategies for reducing inflammation and protecting your brain from further damage.

## The Role of Neuro-Inflammation in Cognitive Dysfunction

Inflammation is a double-edged sword. On one hand, it's a vital part of the body's immune system, helping to fight off infections and heal injuries. However, when inflammation becomes chronic, especially in the brain, it can lead to serious problems. Chronic neuro-inflammation is increasingly recognized as a key factor in various cognitive disorders, including anxiety, depression, ADHD, Alzheimer's disease, and even late-onset ADHD symptoms in adults.

Neuro-inflammation occurs when the brain's immune cells, known as microglia, become overactive. Microglia are responsible for identifying and responding to threats, such as pathogens, toxins, or injury. When they detect a problem, they release inflammatory molecules called cytokines, which help to fight off invaders and repair damage. However, if the microglia are constantly activated— due to ongoing stress, toxin exposure, or other factors—they can start to attack healthy brain cells, leading to widespread inflammation and damage.

This chronic inflammation disrupts normal brain function in several ways:

1. **Impaired Communication Between Neurons:** Inflammation can interfere with the synapses, the connections between neurons, making it harder for them to communicate. This can

lead to symptoms like brain fog, poor memory, and difficulty concentrating.

2. **Disruption of Neurotransmitter Production:** Inflammation can affect the production of neurotransmitters like serotonin, dopamine, and GABA, which are crucial for mood regulation, focus, and overall cognitive function. Low levels of these neurotransmitters can lead to anxiety, depression, and other mood disorders.

3. **Increased Oxidative Stress:** Chronic inflammation generates free radicals, unstable molecules that can damage cells and DNA. This oxidative stress further contributes to neurodegeneration and cognitive decline.

4. **Damage to the Blood-Brain Barrier:** The blood-brain barrier (BBB) is a protective shield that prevents harmful substances from entering the brain. Chronic inflammation can weaken the BBB, allowing toxins, pathogens, and immune cells to infiltrate the brain, exacerbating inflammation and damage.

Given the central role of neuro-inflammation in cognitive dysfunction, it's clear that reducing inflammation is essential for improving brain health. But what causes neuro-inflammation in the first place?

# Common Triggers of Neuro-Inflammation

To effectively reduce neuro-inflammation, we must first understand the common triggers that can set this process in motion. These triggers are often interconnected, creating a vicious cycle that perpetuates inflammation and cognitive decline.

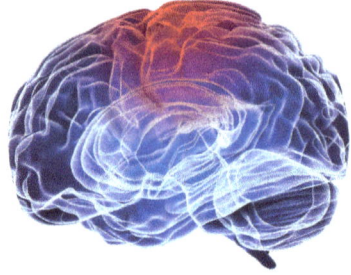

### 1. Toxins and Environmental Exposures

**Heavy Metals:** Exposure to heavy metals like mercury, lead, and aluminum can trigger neuro-inflammation. These metals can accumulate in the brain, where they disrupt neural function and stimulate the release of inflammatory cytokines.

**Pesticides and Chemicals:** Pesticides, herbicides, and other chemicals used in agriculture and industry can enter the body through food, water, and air. There are also lots of chemicals in plastics that can leach into the food if warmed, like a water bottle in a hot car, or food in the microwave. Once inside the body, they can cross the blood-brain barrier and contribute to inflammation.

**Air Pollution:** Fine particulate matter (PM2.5) found in air pollution can reach the brain through the bloodstream, causing oxidative stress and inflammation. Studies have linked long-term exposure to air pollution with increased risks of cognitive decline and neurodegenerative diseases. Chemtrails that are sprayed in the skies are full of nanonized aluminum, barium, and other heavy metals and chemicals. Though hard to avoid, it is important to be aware that it is an issue and could be a source of inhaled toxins.

## 2. Infections

Certain viral infections, such as herpes simplex virus (HSV) and Epstein-Barr virus (EBV), can persist in the body and periodically reactivate, leading to chronic inflammation in the brain.

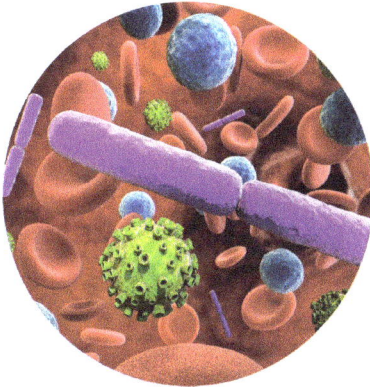

Chronic bacterial infections, such as those caused by Lyme disease, strep, or periodontal disease, can also contribute to neuro-inflammation. These infections can spread to the brain, where they activate microglia and trigger inflammatory responses. Strep can actually target the basal ganglia and cause autism-like symptoms. These symptoms after a strep infection are known as PANDAS.

The gut-brain axis is a bidirectional communication system between the gut and the brain. Infections in the gut, such as small intestinal bacterial overgrowth (SIBO) or parasitic infections, can lead to inflammation in the gut, which in turn triggers inflammation in the brain. The gut and brain mirror each other...if there issues in the gut, there will be issues in the brain and vice versa.

It is very common for people to have low-grade infections for years, even decades, feeding into their chronic symptoms, including those of the brain.

## 3. Chronic Stress

Prolonged emotional stress can lead to chronic activation of the hypothalamic-pituitary-thyroid-adrenal (HPTA) axis, resulting in elevated cortisol levels, Catecholamines (Epinephrine and Norepinephrine) that prepare the body for a "fight or flight" response, inflammatory cytokines, glucose and insulin levels, impaired thyroid function, imbalanced sex hormones, serotonin and dopamine levels, vasopressin, and gastro-intestinal function.

Physical stressors, such as sleep deprivation, overtraining, or chronic pain, can also contribute to neuro-inflammation. These stressors activate the body's stress response, leading to increased production of inflammatory cytokines.

## 4.  Diet and Nutrition

A diet high in refined sugars, unhealthy fats, and processed foods can promote inflammation throughout the body, including the brain. These foods can cause spikes in blood sugar, increase oxidative stress, and disrupt gut health—all of which contribute to neuro-inflammation.  But probably the most overlooked are food sensitivities. When the gut is inflamed and "leaky" it not only will have difficulty digesting proteins into the amino acids the body needs in order to build the proteins it needs for general function and repair, but these partially digested peptides and full proteins can leak through,  getting into the bloodstream and causing an immune response. After constant contact with certain substances, the body can develop a sensitivity, which is detected with IgG food sensitivity testing, NOT traditional allergy tests.  The weaker the mucosal barrier, the more sensitivities one could be experiencing.

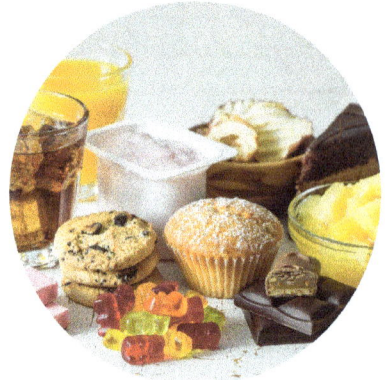

Deficiencies in key nutrients like omega-3 fatty acids, vitamin D, magnesium, and antioxidants can impair the brain's ability to regulate inflammation. Omega-3s, for example, have anti-inflammatory properties that help protect the brain from damage. These deficiencies can be due to lack of consumption, which would be typical in our SAD (standard American diet), or through malabsorption due to the inability to properly digest food and absorb it through an impaired gut lining.

### 5. Sleep Disorders

Sleep apnea, a condition where breathing repeatedly stops and starts during sleep, can lead to hypoxia (low oxygen levels) in the brain. This lack of oxygen triggers inflammation and oxidative stress, contributing to cognitive decline.

Chronic insomnia, or the inability to fall asleep or stay asleep, can exacerbate inflammation by disrupting the brain's natural repair processes. During sleep, the brain clears out waste products and repairs damaged cells. Without adequate sleep, these processes are impaired, leading to increased inflammation.

# The Proverbial Bathtub: Understanding Toxin Accumulation

One useful analogy to understand how neuro-inflammation occurs is to think of your body as a bathtub. Throughout your life, various toxins—whether from environmental exposure, diet, stress, or infections—are continually "poured" into this bathtub. Your body, equipped with natural detoxification pathways, acts as the "drain" that clears out these toxins.

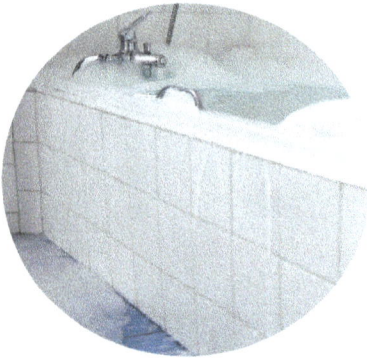

However, when the rate at which toxins enter the bathtub exceeds the body's ability to drain them away, the bathtub begins to fill. Eventually, if too many toxins accumulate and the detox pathways are overwhelmed or blocked, the bathtub will overflow. This overflow is what leads to autoimmunity, neuro-inflammation and cognitive dysfunction.

Toxin accumulation can occur gradually over time or as a result of a significant exposure to harmful substances. Some individuals may have genetic variations that make their detoxification pathways less efficient, leading to a higher risk of toxin buildup and inflammation.

Don't clean out the refrigerator while your house is on fire!

Some people go straight to brain training activities or therapies striving to connect and rewire the brain. However, if the inflammation and other more foundational, root causes aren't being addressed, it is akin to cleaning the refrigerator while your house is on fire. Deal with making sure the immune system is settled and that your body has the essential nutrients before working on rewiring, otherwise those fragile new connections can come apart once therapies cease.

## Strategies to Reduce Neuro-Inflammation

Now that we understand the causes and mechanisms of neuro-inflammation, let's explore practical strategies to reduce inflammation and protect your brain. These strategies focus on removing the sources of inflammation, supporting the body's natural detoxification processes, and enhancing the brain's ability to heal and regenerate.

1. **Remove as many toxins and chemicals as possible** from your environment and replace them with natural ingredients. There may be some things you can't replace or avoid, but reducing the toxic load will help tremendously.

Stop using plastic containers for storing food, especially anything warm or hot, and stop drinking beverages from plastic containers. Start collecting glass containers from grocery shopping, such as jelly jars, juice bottles, and kombucha. There is one brand of kombucha sold at Costco that makes a perfect water bottle.

Try making your own soap and body butter. It is surprisingly simple and there are  hundreds of recipes online. I personally make goat milk soap because goat milk has a similar pH to human skin. The trick with goat milk soap is to freeze it in ice cube trays before preparing so it won't scald when added to the lye.

Buy everything unscented and as dye, color, and chemical free as possible.

2. **Remove any potentially inflammatory foods from your diet**. You may choose to do a food sensitivity test, or simply remove potentially inflammatory foods, such as gluten, dairy, and corn. You can follow an Autoimmune Protocol (AIP) diet for 30 days and then slowly start to reintroduce foods one at a time to see which foods cause a reaction. It is important to note that foods that are being removed need to be done so 100% for a minimum of 10 days. If you find that you have had any of that food, you need to start the 10 days over again as the immune system will have reacted to it, assuming that it is.

The only food that takes longer is gluten. It can take 3-6 months to completely clear the system. This is very tricky because there is hidden gluten EVERYWHERE, even in playdough. If at an Asian restaurant, ask the chef if he adds gluten to the rice, because chances are he does in order for it to be more sticky.

You might want to look in your area for someone who does electrodermal testing for sensitivities, where a probe is placed on specific areas of the hand to determine what things might be causing a problem for the body.

### 3. Adopt an Anti-Inflammatory Diet

Omega-3 fatty acids, particularly EPA and DHA, have powerful anti-inflammatory effects. In fact, high dose DHA after head trauma can prevent or reduce the symptoms of concussion. These fats are found in fatty fish like salmon, sardines, and mackerel, as well as in flaxseeds, chia seeds, and walnuts. Actually, the reason that Omega 3 is in fish in the first place is because they are getting it from algae, the original source. Supplementing with high-quality fish oil or algae sources can also help ensure adequate intake of omega-3s.

Antioxidants neutralize free radicals, reducing oxidative stress and inflammation. Berries (such as blueberries, strawberries, and blackberries), dark leafy greens, and colorful vegetables are excellent sources of antioxidants. Incorporating these foods into your diet can help protect your brain from inflammation.

Reduce or eliminate foods that contribute to inflammation, such as refined sugars, trans fats, and processed foods. These foods can cause spikes in blood sugar, increase oxidative stress, and disrupt gut health, all of which contribute to neuro-inflammation.

Intermittent fasting, or alternating periods of eating and fasting, has been linked to reduced inflammation. Fasting can trigger autophagy, the body's natural process of cleaning out damaged cells and regenerating new ones, which can help reduce oxidative stress and inflammation. Additionally, intermittent fasting may improve metabolic health markers that are often associated with inflammation, such as blood sugar and cholesterol levels.

### 4. Address Infections

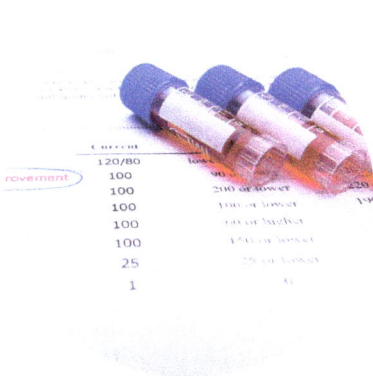

Oftentimes infections are at the bottom of inflammation and need to be appropriately addressed. If you suspect that chronic infections are contributing to your neuro-inflammation, work with a healthcare provider to identify and treat these infections. This may involve antimicrobial treatments, antiviral medications, or herbal remedies. It's important to address these infections early, as they can have long-term effects on brain health if left untreated.

You can see if infections are an issue through your routine blood work, however your average doctor will usually miss this because s/he is not using optimal rangers when looking at the results. If you keep getting told that your bloodwork is normal, yet you are experiencing less than optimal symptoms, then let me take a peek and show you what is driving your symptoms.

### 5. Consider Anti-Inflammatory Supplements

**Curcumin:** Curcumin, the active compound in turmeric, is a potent anti-inflammatory and antioxidant. It has been shown to reduce inflammation in the brain and protect against neurodegenerative diseases. Curcumin supplements are available in various forms, including capsules and powders. To enhance absorption, look for curcumin supplements that contain black pepper extract (piperine), which increases bioavailability.

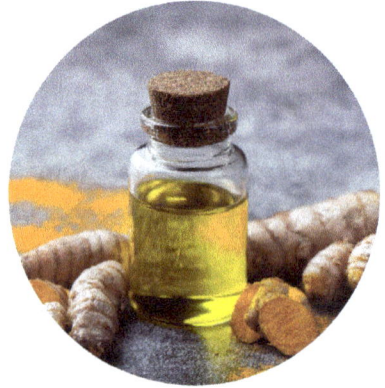

**Resveratrol:** Resveratrol is a polyphenol found in red wine, grapes, and berries. It has anti-inflammatory and neuroprotective properties, making it a valuable supplement for reducing neuro-inflammation. Resveratrol can cross the blood-brain barrier, directly impacting brain health and reducing the risk of cognitive decline.

**Omega-3 Fatty Acids:** As mentioned earlier, omega-3 fatty acids have powerful anti-inflammatory effects. In addition to getting omega-3s from your diet, you may consider taking a high-quality fish oil or algae oil supplement to ensure you're getting an adequate amount.

**Herbal Adaptogens:** Adaptogenic herbs such as ashwagandha, holy basil (tulsi), and astragalus can help modulate the stress response and reduce inflammation. These herbs help the body adapt to stress and balance the immune response, potentially reducing inflammatory markers over time.

**Dietary Polyphenols:** While diet is a common topic in inflammation management, focusing specifically on polyphenols—a type of antioxidant found in foods like berries, tea, dark chocolate, and certain spices—can provide targeted anti-inflammatory effects. Polyphenols can modulate gut microbiota, reduce oxidative stress, and directly inhibit inflammatory pathways.

## Summary

Essentially, you want to remove the sources of inflammation, such as environmental toxins, food sensitivities, endotoxins, and infections, as well as provide the body with things that can help reduce it.

It's important to remember that these changes won't happen overnight. Reducing inflammation and improving brain health is a gradual process that requires consistency and commitment. However, the benefits of taking a proactive approach to neuro-inflammation are profound. Not only can you improve your cognitive function, but you can also enhance your overall quality of life, reduce your risk of chronic diseases, and achieve a greater sense of mental and emotional well-being.

In the next chapter, we'll explore the second step in the 5-step model: detoxification. Detoxifying the body and brain is a crucial step in eliminating the sources of inflammation and creating a clean slate for healing and regeneration. By supporting your body's natural detoxification pathways and reducing your exposure to toxins, you can further protect your brain and optimize its function.

# 3

# Step 2
# – Detoxification

## The Importance of Detoxification for Brain Health

Detoxification is a critical step in optimizing brain health and function. Just as you wouldn't expect a car to run smoothly if its fuel lines were clogged with debris, you can't expect your brain to operate at peak performance if it's burdened with toxins. Over time, our bodies accumulate various toxins from the environment, food, water, and even the air we breathe. These toxins can interfere with brain function, contributing to symptoms like brain fog, anxiety, poor focus, and even long-term cognitive decline.

The detoxification process is the body's way of clearing out these harmful substances, allowing your brain to function more efficiently. However, detoxification is not just about flushing out toxins—it's about supporting the body's natural processes, enhancing its ability to eliminate waste, and creating an environment in which the brain can heal and thrive.

In this chapter, we'll explore the importance of detoxification for brain health, the sources of toxins that affect the brain, and practical strategies for effectively detoxifying the body and brain.

# Understanding the Body's Detoxification System

Before diving into the specifics of how to detoxify the brain, it's essential to understand how the body's detoxification system works. The body has a complex, multi-organ system designed to eliminate toxins and waste products. The primary organs involved in detoxification include:

1. **The Liver:** The liver is the body's main detoxification organ. It processes toxins and waste products from the blood, converting them into forms that can be safely excreted from the body. The liver's detoxification process occurs in technically 4 phases:

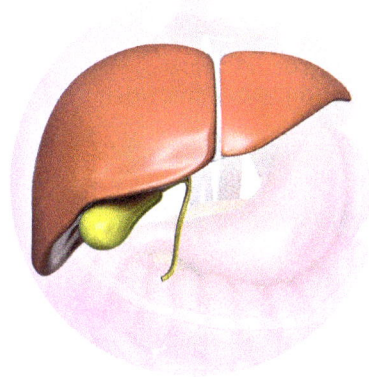

**Phase 0 Detoxification:** This phase involves the transport and absorption of toxins into cells, particularly liver cells, where detoxification occurs. Various transport proteins regulate the entry of toxins across cell membranes, determining how much of a toxin is absorbed for further processing and how much remains in circulation. Phase 0 is crucial in managing the detoxification load on the liver and other organs, ensuring that the body's detox pathways are not overwhelmed.

**Phase I Detoxification:** In this phase, the liver utilizes a group of enzymes, primarily from the cytochrome P450 family, to modify toxins into more reactive intermediate metabolites. These reactions typically involve oxidation, reduction, or hydrolysis, transforming fat-soluble toxins into more water-soluble forms. However, this process can produce free radicals and other reactive oxygen species (ROS) as by-products, which can be harmful if not neutralized by antioxidants.

**Phase II Detoxification:** Following Phase I, the liver continues to process the intermediate metabolites by conjugating them with molecules such as glutathione, sulfate, or glucuronic acid. This conjugation process makes the metabolites more water-soluble and less reactive, facilitating their safe excretion from the body. Phase II detoxification plays a crucial role in reducing the toxicity of intermediate metabolites and preparing them for elimination.

**Phase III Detoxification:** The final phase of detoxification involves the transport of conjugated toxins out of the cells and into the bile or urine for excretion. Efflux transporters actively pump these water-soluble, conjugated toxins from liver cells into the bile, which is then released into the intestines, or into the bloodstream for renal excretion via urine. Phase III ensures the efficient elimination of toxins from the body, preventing their reabsorption and promoting overall detoxification.

2. **The Kidneys:** The kidneys filter waste products and excess fluids from the blood, excreting them as urine. They play a critical role in maintaining the body's fluid balance and eliminating water-soluble toxins.

In addition to filtering waste and excess fluids, the kidneys regulate electrolyte levels, such as sodium, potassium, and calcium, which are vital for nerve function, muscle contraction, and overall cellular health. They also maintain acid-base balance by excreting hydrogen ions and reabsorbing bicarbonate, ensuring the blood's pH remains within a healthy range. This precise regulation of fluids and electrolytes helps prevent dehydration, supports cardiovascular health, and facilitates the elimination of water-soluble toxins and metabolic by-products, safeguarding the body from the buildup of harmful substances.

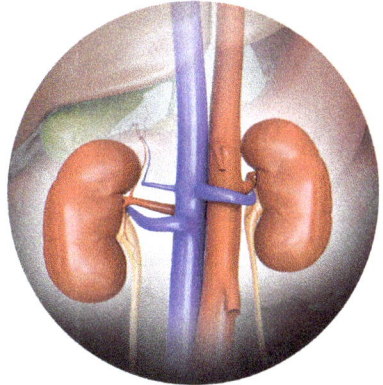

3. **The Colon:** The colon, or large intestine, plays a crucial role in detoxification and the elimination of solid waste from the body. In addition to absorbing water and electrolytes from indigestible food matter, the colon also serves as a critical site for the removal of toxins and waste products processed by the liver.

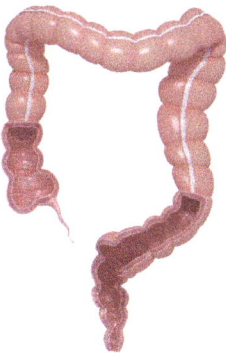

Bile, which contains conjugated toxins from liver detoxification, is secreted into the intestines and eventually reaches the colon. Here, fiber binds to these toxins, aiding their incorporation into stool.

The colon's microbial flora also contributes to detoxification by breaking down certain compounds and maintaining a healthy gut barrier, preventing the reabsorption of toxins back into the bloodstream. Efficient colon function is therefore essential for the complete elimination of waste and for maintaining the body's overall detoxification process.

4. **The Lymphatic System:** The lymphatic system, a crucial component of the body's detoxification network, not only removes waste and toxins from tissues but also plays a vital role in maintaining immune function and fluid balance. By transporting lymph—a fluid rich in white blood cells, proteins, and waste products—through a network of lymph vessels and nodes, the lymphatic system captures and filters out toxins, bacteria, and other harmful substances.

Lymph nodes act as filtration centers, trapping pathogens and facilitating their destruction by immune cells. Additionally, the lymphatic system helps drain excess fluids from tissues, preventing swelling and promoting the efficient removal of cellular waste. A well-functioning lymphatic system supports overall detoxification, ensuring that toxins are effectively cleared from the body and do not accumulate in tissues.

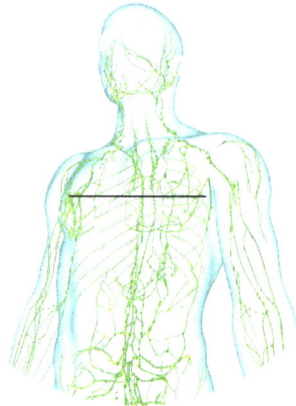

5. **The Skin:** The skin, the body's largest organ, serves as a vital component of the detoxification process, primarily through the action of sweat glands. As the body heats up, sweat glands produce sweat, which not only helps regulate body temperature but also assists in excreting toxins and metabolic waste products, such as urea, ammonia, and heavy metals. This process aids in reducing the toxic burden on internal

organs, such as the liver and kidneys, by providing an additional route for waste elimination. Moreover, regular sweating through activities like exercise, saunas, or hot baths can enhance the skin's detoxification capacity by stimulating circulation and opening pores, allowing for more effective removal of toxins. Thus, the skin acts as a dynamic barrier and detoxification organ, playing a crucial role in maintaining overall health and supporting the body's natural cleansing processes.

6. **The Lungs:** The lungs play a vital role in the body's detoxification processes by expelling carbon dioxide, a waste product of cellular metabolism, from the bloodstream. Every time we exhale, the lungs remove carbon dioxide and other volatile substances, including toxins and pollutants that have been inhaled. This process is essential for maintaining the body's pH balance and preventing the buildup of harmful gasses in the blood. The lungs also act as a first line of defense against airborne toxins and pathogens by trapping them in mucus and expelling them through coughing or sneezing. Additionally, the deep breathing exercises often recommended for detoxification practices, such as yoga or meditation, help enhance lung capacity, improve oxygen exchange, and support the release of toxins, further contributing to the body's natural detoxification pathways. By maintaining healthy lung function and practicing mindful breathing, we can

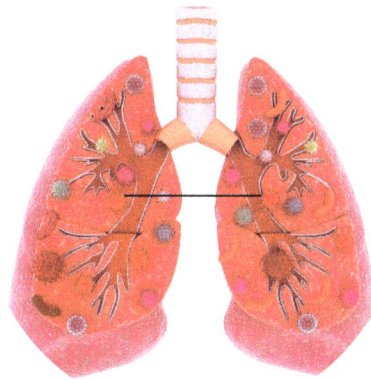

support the lungs' role in detoxifying the body and promoting overall health.

7. **The Brain's Glymphatic System:** The brain has its own unique detoxification system called the glymphatic system. This system is most active during sleep and helps clear out waste products, such as beta-amyloid (a protein linked to Alzheimer's disease), from the brain. The glymphatic system relies on cerebrospinal fluid (CSF) to flush out toxins and metabolic waste, making sleep a critical component of brain detoxification. Massaging the nodes around the neck before bed can help activate the glymphatic system and increase drainage.

These systems work together to ensure that toxins are efficiently removed from the body. However, when these systems become overwhelmed or impaired—due to factors like poor diet, lack of exercise, chronic stress, or genetic predispositions—toxins can accumulate, leading to a range of health problems, including cognitive dysfunction.

# Sources of Toxins That Affect Brain Health

To effectively detoxify the body and brain, it's important to understand where toxins come from and how they enter the body. The following are some of the most common sources of toxins that can affect brain health, many which we have already discussed in the previous chapter on inflammation :

### 1. Heavy Metals

**Mercury:** Mercury is a toxic heavy metal that can enter the body through seafood (especially large fish like tuna and swordfish), dental amalgam fillings, and certain industrial processes. Particularly in its organic form as methylmercury, it is a potent neurotoxin that can significantly affect the brain. It readily crosses the blood-brain barrier, where it accumulates and disrupts neural function by binding to proteins and enzymes critical for normal brain activity. Mercury exposure can lead to oxidative stress, inflammation, and interference with neurotransmitter systems, particularly those involving glutamate and gamma-aminobutyric acid (GABA), which are essential for cognitive function and mood regulation. The damage caused by mercury can impair memory, attention, and motor skills, and is especially harmful during developmental stages, potentially leading to long-term cognitive and behavioral deficits.

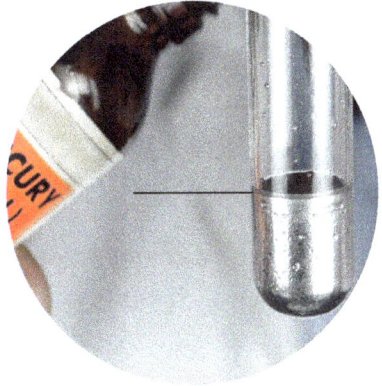

Check out the YouTube video clip "smoking teeth" that shows with special cameras the continual off gassing of amalgam fillings.  It is especially important to remove these fillings at least  months before pregnancy to prevent transmission into the fetus.

**Lead:** Lead exposure, often resulting from sources like old paint, contaminated water from lead pipes, and industrial pollution, poses a severe threat to the nervous system. They can also be found in the glaze used in dishes, especially in other countries, and machinery used to make candy in Mexico.

Once absorbed, lead can cross the blood-brain barrier and accumulate in the brain, where it disrupts neural development and function. It interferes with neurotransmitter release, synapse formation, and myelination, all crucial for normal cognitive function. In children, whose brains are still developing, lead exposure is particularly damaging, leading to cognitive deficits such as reduced IQ, attention disorders, learning difficulties, and behavioral issues.

**Aluminum:** Aluminum, commonly found in cookware, food packaging, some antacids, deodorants, and as an adjuvant in most vaccines, can pose a significant risk to brain health when exposure levels are high. It is also cited as a primary component in "chemtrails."

While the body can excrete small amounts of aluminum, excessive exposure can lead to its accumulation in the brain, where it disrupts neurological function. Aluminum can impair the blood-brain barrier, promote oxidative stress, and induce inflammation, which are all factors linked to the development of neurodegenerative diseases like Alzheimer's. Chronic aluminum exposure has been associated with the formation of

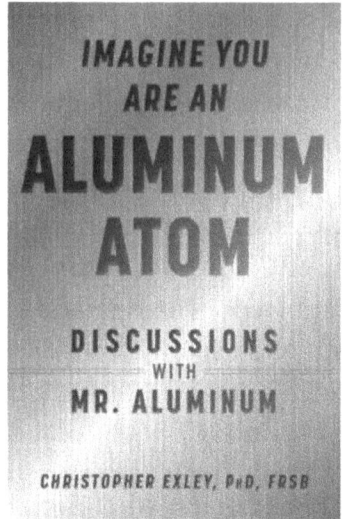

IMAGINE YOU ARE AN **ALUMINUM ATOM**

**DISCUSSIONS** WITH **MR. ALUMINUM**

CHRISTOPHER EXLEY, PhD, FRSB

amyloid plaques and neurofibrillary tangles, hallmarks of Alzheimer's disease, making it crucial to minimize exposure to this metal to protect brain health.

A great book to read on this topic is "Imagine You Were an Aluminum Atom" by Christopher Exley.

### 2. Environmental Chemicals

**Pesticides:** Pesticides used in agriculture can contaminate food and water supplies, posing significant risks to human health. Many pesticides are neurotoxic, meaning they can interfere with the normal functioning of the nervous system. These chemicals can cross the blood-brain barrier and accumulate in neural tissue, where they disrupt neurotransmitter function, induce oxidative stress, and cause neuronal damage. Chronic exposure to neurotoxic pesticides has been linked to cognitive issues such as memory loss, reduced attention span, and impaired learning abilities. Long-term exposure, even at low levels, can increase the risk of developing neurological conditions such as Parkinson's disease, making it important to reduce pesticide exposure through organic food choices and proper washing of fruits and vegetables.

**Bisphenol A (BPA):** Bisphenol A (BPA) is a chemical commonly used in the production of plastics, including water bottles, food containers, and the lining of canned foods. BPA can leach into food and beverages, especially when containers are heated or damaged, leading to ingestion and accumulation in the body. BPA is known to be an endocrine disruptor, mimicking estrogen and interfering with hormone signaling pathways, which can impact brain development and function.

Studies have linked BPA exposure to cognitive problems, including impaired memory, learning difficulties, and altered behavior, particularly in children and fetuses, whose brains are still developing. Given its potential to disrupt hormonal balance and affect cognitive health, minimizing exposure to BPA by opting for BPA-free products and avoiding plastic containers for hot or acidic foods is crucial.

**Phthalates:** Phthalates are chemicals used to make plastics more flexible and are commonly found in a wide range of products, including personal care items like shampoos and lotions, food packaging, and household products. These chemicals are known endocrine disruptors, meaning they interfere with the body's hormonal systems by mimicking or blocking natural hormones, particularly those involved in reproductive and developmental processes. Phthalate exposure has been associated with cognitive and behavioral issues, especially in children. Studies suggest that these chemicals can affect brain development, leading to problems with attention, learning, and behavior. Reducing exposure to phthalates by choosing phthalate-free personal care products, avoiding plastic food containers, and opting for fresh, unpackaged foods can help mitigate their potential impact on health.

### 3. Airborne Toxins

**Air Pollution:** Air pollution, particularly fine particulate matter (PM2.5), poses a significant threat to brain health. These tiny particles can penetrate deep into the lungs and enter the bloodstream, where they travel to the brain, crossing the blood-brain barrier. Once in the brain, PM2.5 can cause inflammation, oxidative stress, and neuronal damage. Long-term exposure to air pollution has been linked to cognitive decline, including memory loss and decreased attention span, and is associated with an increased risk of neurodegenerative diseases such as Alzheimer's and Parkinson's. The chronic inflammatory response triggered by these pollutants can exacerbate brain aging and neurodegenerative processes, highlighting the importance of reducing exposure to air pollution for maintaining cognitive health.

**Mold:** Mold exposure, particularly in damp or water-damaged buildings, can be a root cause of many chronic, hard-to-treat conditions. Mold growth in these environments can release mycotoxins—potent toxins that can easily be inhaled or absorbed through the skin. These mycotoxins pose serious health risks, leading to a wide range of symptoms, including respiratory problems, immune suppression, and cognitive dysfunction.

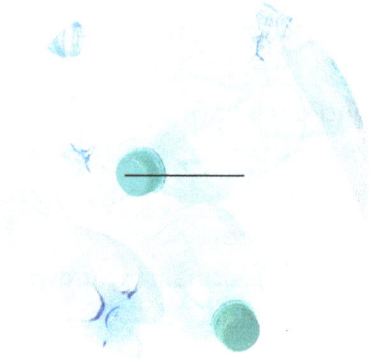

The neurotoxic effects of mycotoxins can cause memory loss, brain fog, and difficulty concentrating, contributing to long-term neurological issues. Moreover, mycotoxins can exacerbate chronic inflammatory responses and weaken the immune system, making the body more vulnerable to infections and other health challenges. Addressing mold exposure is crucial for preventing these extensive health impacts and maintaining overall well-being.

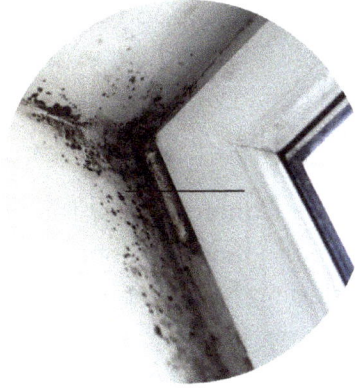

## 4. Food and Water Contaminants

**Pesticides and Herbicides:** Pesticides and herbicides used in conventional agriculture are common contaminants in food and water supplies. These chemicals, designed to kill pests and weeds, can also disrupt human health, particularly affecting the nervous system. Many pesticides are neurotoxic, potentially leading to cognitive issues such as memory problems, attention deficits, and developmental delays, especially in children.

Herbicides like glyphosate have been linked to disruptions in gut health, which can indirectly affect brain function. To reduce exposure, opting for organic foods that are free from synthetic pesticides and herbicides is recommended. Additionally, filtering drinking water can help remove these contaminants, as well as other harmful substances that may leach into water supplies from agricultural runoff.

**Food Additives:** Many processed foods contain a variety of additives, preservatives, artificial colors, and flavors that may negatively impact brain health. For example, monosodium glutamate (MSG), commonly used to enhance flavor, can act as an excitotoxin, potentially overstimulating brain cells to the point of damage or death. Similarly, artificial sweeteners like aspartame have been linked to neurotoxicity, potentially leading to headaches, mood changes, and even cognitive decline. To support detoxification and protect brain health, it's beneficial to reduce consumption of processed foods and focus on a diet rich in whole, unprocessed foods that provide essential nutrients without harmful additives.

**Water Contaminants:** Tap water can harbor a range of contaminants, including heavy metals like lead, chlorine, fluoride, and even pharmaceutical residues from improperly disposed medications. Lead, in particular, is a potent neurotoxin that can impair cognitive function and development, while chlorine and fluoride, though added for disinfection and dental health, respectively, may also pose health risks in high amounts. Pharmaceutical residues in water can disrupt endocrine function and potentially affect brain health. Using a high-quality water filter that can remove these contaminants is crucial for reducing toxic load and supporting overall detoxification processes in the body.

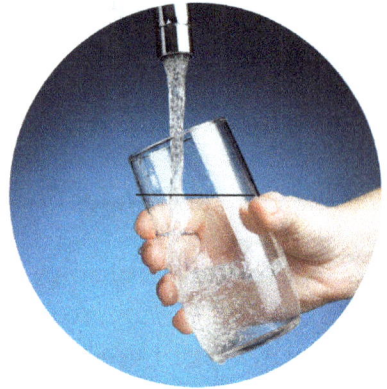

Fluoride is a known neurotoxin and should NOT be consumed. It is typically added to city water. It is important to go to your city's website in order to determine if fluoride has been added where you live. More than likely it has. Fluoride is extremely difficult to filter out of the water and you need a special filter that may only get a percentage of it. Berkey water filters has an optional fluoride filter, the efficacy is debatable, but it seems to get at least 35%. A great book to read on this topic is "The Fluoride Deception" by Christopher Bryson.

### 5. Personal Care and Household Products

**Cosmetics and Skincare Products:** Many personal care products, including cosmetics, lotions, and skincare items, contain chemicals like parabens, phthalates, and synthetic fragrances that can be absorbed through the skin. These chemicals are known endocrine disruptors, which means they can interfere with hormone function and potentially contribute to toxin buildup in the body. Parabens, for example, are preservatives that have been linked to hormone disruption and may have carcinogenic effects.

**Cleaning Products:** Household cleaning products often contain harsh chemicals that can release volatile organic compounds (VOCs) into the air, contributing to indoor air pollution and potential neurotoxicity. VOCs, such as formaldehyde and ammonia, can irritate the respiratory system, cause headaches, and may even lead to long-term neurological effects with prolonged exposure. Additionally, certain disinfectants and antibacterial agents, like triclosan, have been linked to hormone disruption and may contribute to microbial resistance. Switching to natural or homemade cleaning products, which use safer ingredients like vinegar, baking soda, and essential oils, can help reduce toxic exposure, improve indoor air quality, and protect brain health.

### 6. Medications and Pharmaceuticals

**Over-the-Counter Medications:** While over-the-counter medications are easily accessible and widely used for minor ailments, some can have toxic effects, particularly when used frequently or in high doses. For instance, acetaminophen (Tylenol) is a common pain reliever and fever reducer, but it can be toxic to the liver, especially with prolonged use or overdose. Since the liver is a primary organ for detoxification, impairing its function can lead to an accumulation of toxins in the body, increasing the risk of various health issues, including neurotoxicity. It is essential to use such medications sparingly and under medical supervision to avoid potential toxicity and support the body's natural detox processes.

**Prescription Drugs:** Certain prescription medications, particularly those used to treat mood disorders and anxiety, can have side effects that impact brain health. Benzodiazepines, for example, are commonly prescribed for anxiety and insomnia but have been linked to cognitive decline with long-term use, potentially affecting memory, concentration, and learning abilities. Some antipsychotic drugs and antidepressants can also alter neurotransmitter levels in the brain, potentially leading to side effects that impair cognitive function.

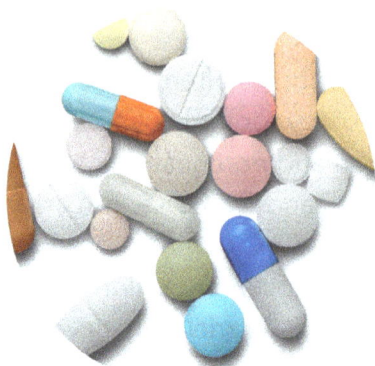

Patients and healthcare providers must carefully weigh the benefits and risks of these medications, considering alternatives where possible, and take steps to mitigate side effects that could impact brain health and overall well-being. If you are taking such medications, it is critical to work with your physician if you are trying to wean yourself off of them, as some can cause serious problems if suddenly removed.

Understanding these sources of toxins is crucial for taking proactive steps to reduce your exposure and support your body's detoxification processes.

# Supporting the Body's Natural Detoxification Processes

Effective detoxification is not about taking drastic measures or following extreme detox diets. Instead, it's about supporting the body's natural detoxification processes, enhancing the organs and systems responsible for eliminating toxins, and making sustainable lifestyle changes that reduce your overall toxin burden.

Here are some practical strategies to support your body's natural detoxification processes:

• **Enhance Liver Function**

**Eat Detoxifying Foods:** Certain foods are known to support liver function and enhance detoxification. These include cruciferous vegetables (e.g., broccoli, cauliflower, Brussels sprouts), garlic, onions, beets, and leafy greens. These foods provide the liver with the nutrients it needs to process and eliminate toxins effectively.

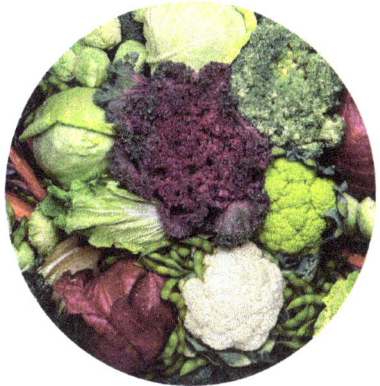

**Incorporate Herbal Support:** Herbs like milk thistle, dandelion root, and turmeric have been traditionally used to support liver health. Milk thistle contains silymarin, a compound that protects liver cells from damage and supports regeneration. Dandelion root is a natural diuretic that helps flush out toxins, while turmeric has powerful anti-inflammatory and antioxidant properties that protect the liver.  If it's bitter, it is probably helpful.

**Limit Alcohol Consumption:** Alcohol is metabolized by the liver and can be particularly taxing on this organ. Limiting alcohol consumption—or avoiding it altogether—can significantly reduce the liver's toxic load and support detoxification.

**Do coffee enemas**:  Coffee enemas stimulate the liver to produce more bile and enhance glutathione production, a powerful antioxidant that aids in detoxification and neutralizes free radicals, thereby reducing oxidative stress. They may also improve digestion and bowel function by stimulating peristalsis and alleviating constipation, which can help cleanse the colon of accumulated waste and toxins. Enemas can  enhance mental clarity and energy levels by promoting the removal of toxins from the body, potentially alleviating symptoms like brain fog and fatigue.

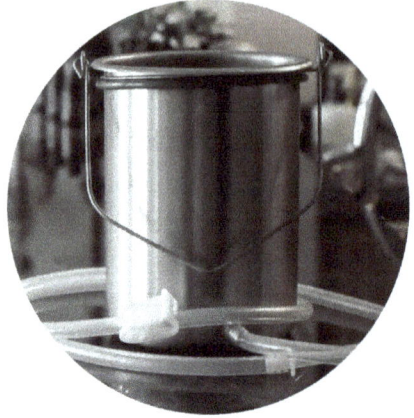

## Support Kidney Health

**Stay Hydrated:** Drinking plenty of water is essential for kidney function. Water helps flush out toxins and waste products, preventing them from accumulating in the body. Aim to drink at least 8-10 glasses of water per day, and consider increasing your intake if you're physically active or live in a hot climate.

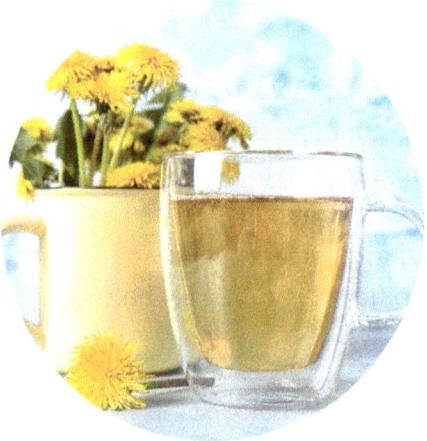

**Eat Kidney-Supportive Foods:** Certain foods and herbs are particularly beneficial for maintaining kidney health and supporting their detoxification function. Foods like cranberries, blueberries, and celery are rich in antioxidants and have natural diuretic properties that help cleanse the kidneys and support urinary tract health. Cranberries, in particular, are well-known for their ability to prevent urinary tract infections (UTIs) by preventing bacteria from adhering to the urinary tract walls, reducing the risk of infections that can place additional strain on the kidneys.

Additionally, specific herbs like dandelion root, nettle leaf, parsley, astragalus, and juniper berry are renowned for their kidney-supportive properties. Juniper berry, in particular, is a potent diuretic that promotes increased urine output, helping to flush out excess fluids, salts, and toxins from the kidneys. It also has natural antiseptic properties that can help prevent infections in the urinary tract. Dandelion root acts as a gentle diuretic, while nettle leaf is rich in vitamins and minerals that support kidney function and reduce inflammation. Parsley aids in the elimination of excess fluids, and astragalus protects kidney cells and enhances overall kidney function. Incorporating these foods and herbs into the diet can help maintain healthy kidney function, enhance detoxification, and support overall well-being.

**Avoid Excessive Sodium:** High sodium intake in the form of table salt can increase blood pressure and place additional stress on the kidneys.  Replace the highly processed table salt  with celtic sea salt or pink salt (Real Salt is my favorite), which will actually normalize blood pressure as it contains up to 85 trace minerals necessary for appropriate  body function.  Reducing your intake of processed foods, which are often high in sodium, and using herbs and spices to flavor your meals instead of salt can also help protect your kidneys.

## Optimize Gut Health

Optimizing gut health is crucial for maintaining brain health, as the gut-brain axis plays a key role in regulating mood, cognition, and overall neurological function. A healthy gut microbiome supports proper digestion and detoxification, preventing harmful substances from reaching the brain and causing neuroinflammation or cognitive decline.

**Increase Fiber Intake:** Fiber is essential for healthy digestion and regular bowel movements, which are critical for eliminating toxins from the body. Foods rich in fiber include fruits, vegetables, whole grains, legumes, and seeds. Fiber binds to toxins in the digestive tract and helps remove them through stool.

**Incorporate Probiotics and Prebiotics:** Probiotics are beneficial bacteria that support a healthy gut microbiome, while prebiotics are fibers that feed these bacteria. Bacteria excrete things, and those things can either help or hinder the body and brain. There are hundreds of different strains of bacteria, most of which aren't yet identified or well understood. Carefully choosing probiotics that target what you want is important.

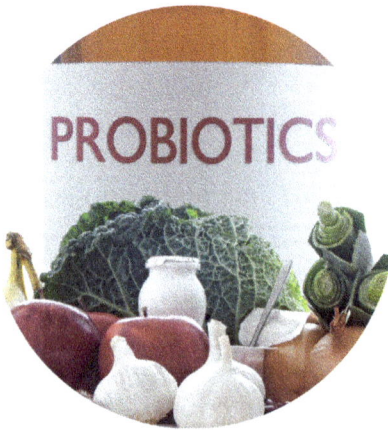

In order to increase general diversity in the gut, fermented foods like yogurt, kefir, sauerkraut, and kimchi are excellent sources of probiotics, whole foods like garlic, onions, and bananas provide prebiotics which feed those microbes. A healthy gut microbiome is essential for efficient detoxification and overall brain health. Making your own fermented foods is a lot easier than it seems.

**Consider Periodic Fasting:** Intermittent fasting or periodic fasting can give the digestive system a break and enhance the body's natural detoxification processes. Fasting stimulates autophagy, a process in which the body breaks down and recycles damaged cells and proteins, helping to clear out toxins and reduce inflammation.Promote Lymphatic Drainage

## Promote Lymphatic Drainage

Engaging in regular exercise, such as walking, jogging, yoga, and rebounding (jumping on a mini-trampoline), is an effective way to stimulate the lymphatic system and promote the flow of lymph, which helps remove toxins from the body. In addition to physical activity, other practices like dry brushing and lymphatic massage can further support lymphatic drainage and detoxification. Dry brushing involves using a natural bristle brush to gently stroke the skin in the direction of the heart, which can enhance circulation and stimulate the lymphatic system, aiding in the elimination of toxins through the skin. Incorporating lymphatic drainage massage, either by a trained therapist or through self-massage techniques, can also encourage the movement of lymph and facilitate the removal of toxins, contributing to overall detoxification and improved health.

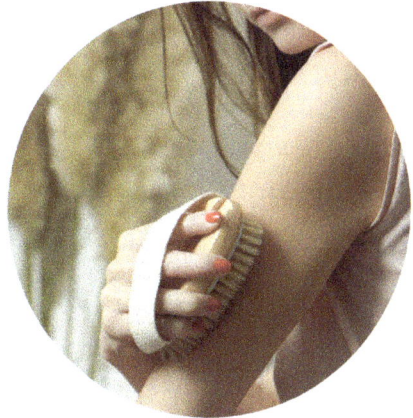

## Sweat It Out

**Use a Sauna:** Regular use of a sauna, particularly an infrared sauna, can enhance detoxification by promoting sweating. Sweating helps eliminate toxins through the skin, including heavy metals, phthalates, and other environmental toxins. Start with short sessions and gradually increase the time spent in the sauna as your body becomes accustomed to the heat.  Quick tip…if you suspect heavy metals, midway through your sauna session, wipe yourself down with a small towel and put it outside of the sauna so the metals don't get reabsorbed back into the heat of the sauna, which will be quickly absorbed in your skin.

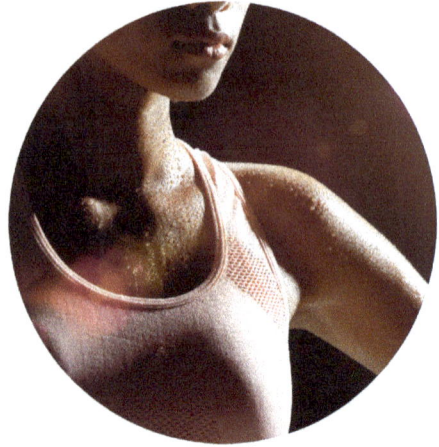

**Engage in Vigorous Exercise:** Vigorous exercise, such as high-intensity interval training (HIIT), can also promote sweating and detoxification. In addition to its benefits for the lymphatic system and cardiovascular health, exercise-induced sweating helps remove toxins from the body.

**Stay Hydrated:** After sweating, it's important to rehydrate with plenty of water to support kidney function and prevent dehydration. Adding electrolytes to your water can help replenish minerals lost through sweat.

## Detox Your Environment

**Improve Indoor Air Quality:** Use air purifiers to reduce indoor air pollution, and regularly ventilate your home to allow fresh air to circulate. Houseplants like spider plants, snake plants, and peace lilies can also help improve indoor air quality by absorbing toxins.

**Choose Non-Toxic Cleaning Products:** Opt for natural, non-toxic cleaning products to reduce your exposure to harmful chemicals. You can also make your own cleaning solutions using ingredients like vinegar, baking soda, and essential oils.

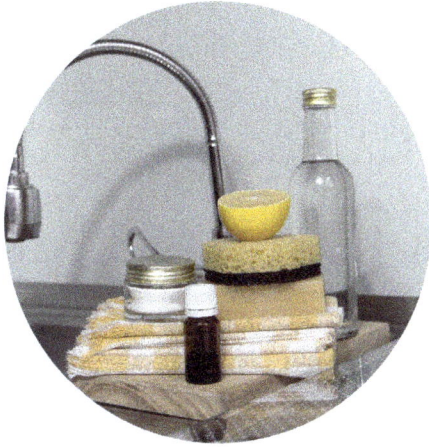

**Filter Your Water:** Use a high-quality water filter to remove contaminants like heavy metals, chlorine, and fluoride from your drinking water. A reverse osmosis filter is particularly effective for removing a wide range of toxins.

**Avoid Plastic Containers:** Store food and beverages in glass or stainless-steel containers instead of plastic, which can leach chemicals like BPA and phthalates into your food. If you must use plastic, choose BPA-free options and avoid heating food in plastic containers.

## Support Brain Detoxification with Sleep

**Prioritize Quality Sleep:** As mentioned earlier, the brain's glymphatic system is most active during sleep. Prioritizing quality sleep is essential for effective brain detoxification. Aim for 7-9 hours of sleep per night, and establish a relaxing bedtime routine to improve sleep quality.

**Sleep on Your Side:** Research suggests that sleeping on your side, rather than on your back or stomach, may enhance the glymphatic system's ability to clear waste from the brain. This sleeping position is believed to facilitate the flow of cerebrospinal fluid, which helps remove toxins from the brain.

You might also try sleeping with the head of the bed raised about 5%. This helps that glymphatic drainage as you sleep. You can put something under the legs to raise it, sleep on a few fat pillows to cause you to be elevated, or get a bed that you can adjust. We have a bed from Ikea that is manually adjustable, much like a lawn chair.

**Practice Sleep Hygiene:** Keep your bedroom dark, quiet, and cool, and avoid screens an hour before bed to support the production of melatonin. Melatonin not only regulates sleep but also has antioxidant properties that help protect the brain from oxidative stress and inflammation.

# The Role of Targeted Detoxification Protocols

In some cases, especially if you suspect a high level of toxin exposure or if you have specific health concerns, it may be beneficial to follow a targeted detoxification protocol. These protocols are designed to address specific toxins or health issues and should be tailored to your individual needs.

Here are a few examples of targeted detoxification protocols:

## Heavy Metal Detoxification

**Chelation Therapy:** Chelation therapy involves the use of chelating agents, such as EDTA or DMSA, to bind to heavy metals and facilitate their excretion from the body. This therapy should only be done under the supervision of a healthcare provider, as it can have side effects and may require supplementation with essential minerals to prevent deficiencies. This might be done orally or through IV chelation.

**Natural Chelators:** Certain foods and supplements can also help remove heavy metals from the body. These natural chelators can be incorporated into your diet or taken as supplements. For example, cilantro is known to mobilize certain metals, like mercury, and chlorella is known to bind to them to support their excretion. Other popular binders are apple pectin, zeolite (specifically for positively charged metals like aluminum), and bentonite clay.  Activated charcoal binds to both toxins and minerals, so this binder is usually reserved for acute illnesses or short-term binding. There are specialty labs that have created binders by blending a variety of natural items.  If you are interested, you can check out the links at the end of this book.

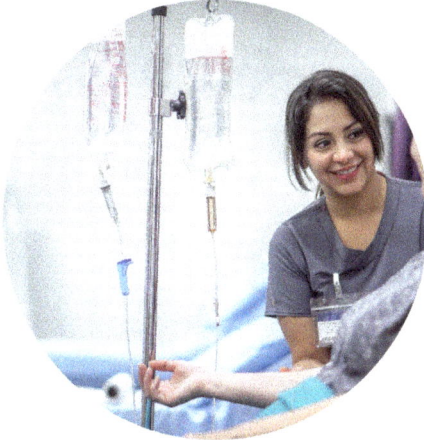

One thing to note…metals take the binding sites of minerals, so flooding the body with minerals is important in order to help kick the metals out of the binding sites and prevent them from re-docking.

## Liver Detoxification Protocols

**Glutathione Supplementation:** Glutathione is the body's most powerful antioxidant and plays a crucial role in liver detoxification. Supplementing with glutathione or its precursors, such as N-acetylcysteine (NAC), can support the liver's ability to detoxify harmful substances.

Something to note, taking glutathione orally has a half-life of 7 minutes.  Therefore, helping the body to increase its own production is a helpful addition. Lifewave®'s Glutathione phototherapy patch can help the body to produce up to 300% more of its natural glutathione and sustain it. See link at the end of this book.

**Liver Cleanses:** Some people choose to do a liver cleanse, which typically involves a short-term diet focused on liver-supportive foods, along with specific supplements or herbal teas. Liver cleanses are meant to give the liver a break from processing toxins and allow it to regenerate. I have a couple of great protocols for liver cleanses if this is something that you are interested in.

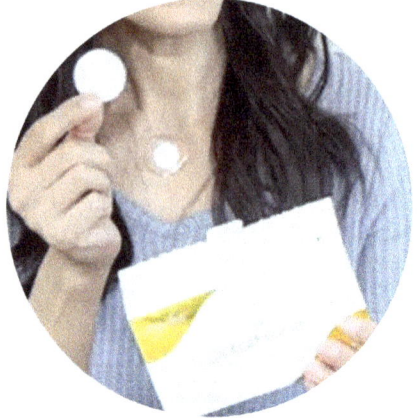

**Gut Reset Programs:** A gut reset program typically involves eliminating inflammatory foods, taking probiotics and prebiotics, and incorporating gut-healing nutrients like L-glutamine, aloe vera, and bone broth in order to rebuild the mucosal lining. This type of program is designed to restore gut health, reduce inflammation, and support the body's natural detoxification processes.

**Parasite Cleanses:** Parasite cleanses are designed to eliminate parasitic infections from the gut. These cleanses often involve the use of antiparasitic herbs like wormwood, black walnut, and cloves, along with a diet that starves parasites of their food sources (e.g., sugar and processed foods).

# Conclusion: The Path to a Cleaner, Healthier Brain

Detoxification is a vital step in optimizing brain health and function. By reducing your toxic burden, supporting your body's natural detox processes, and making sustainable lifestyle changes, you can create an environment in which your brain can thrive.

Remember, detoxification is not about quick fixes or extreme measures—it's about making thoughtful, long-term changes that support your body's ability to cleanse itself and function at its best.

You should periodically engage in detoxifying your body because we are in constant contact with many toxins.

By incorporating the strategies outlined in this chapter, you'll be well on your way to achieving a cleaner, healthier brain, free from the burden of toxins that can cloud your thoughts, disrupt your focus, and compromise your well-being.

In the next chapter, we'll explore the third step in the 5-step model: nourishing the brain. Once you've cleared out the toxins and reduced inflammation, it's time to focus on providing your brain and body with the essential nutrients it needs to repair, regenerate, and function at its peak.

# 4

## Step 3
## - Nourishing the Brain

### Introduction: The Power of Nutrition in Brain Health

After addressing inflammation and detoxification, the next critical step in optimizing brain health is nourishing the brain. Imagine your brain as a highly sophisticated engine. Just as a high-performance car needs premium fuel to run at its best, your brain requires specific nutrients to function optimally. When provided with the right nutrients, your brain can repair itself, create new neural connections, and maintain peak cognitive performance. Conversely, a lack of essential nutrients can lead to cognitive decline, mood disturbances, and other neurological issues.

In this chapter, we'll explore the key nutrients that support brain health, how to incorporate them into your diet, and additional strategies to ensure your brain is getting the nourishment it needs. By the end of this chapter, you'll have a comprehensive understanding of how to fuel your brain for optimal function and longevity.

# The Role of Key Nutrients in Brain Function

The brain is an energy-intensive organ, consuming approximately 20% of the body's total energy supply despite making up only about 2% of body weight. To perform its complex functions—such as processing information, regulating emotions, and coordinating movement—the brain relies on a steady supply of essential nutrients. These nutrients not only provide energy but also serve as building blocks for neurotransmitters, protect against oxidative stress, and support neuroplasticity (the brain's ability to adapt and change).

Let's explore the key nutrients that are essential for brain health:

## Omega-3 Fatty Acids

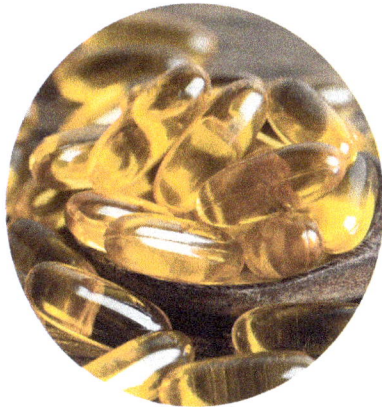

Omega-3 fatty acids, particularly docosahexaenoic acid (DHA) and eicosapentaenoic acid (EPA), are among the most important nutrients for brain health. DHA is a major structural component of the brain, making up about 40% of the polyunsaturated fatty acids in the brain and 60% in the retina of the eye. EPA, while present in smaller amounts, plays a crucial role in reducing inflammation and supporting overall brain function.

Research has shown that DHA is essential for brain development and function throughout life. It supports the structure of cell membranes in the brain, enhances communication between neurons, and promotes neurogenesis (the formation of new neurons). EPA, on the other hand, has been shown to reduce symptoms of depression and anxiety by modulating the production of inflammatory cytokines and influencing serotonin function.

The best dietary sources of DHA and EPA are fatty fish such as salmon, mackerel, sardines, and anchovies. For those who do not consume fish, algal oil is a plant-based source of DHA. Omega-3 supplements, such as fish oil or krill oil, are also effective ways to ensure adequate intake.  A typical dose is 1,000-2,000 mg of combined DHA and EPA daily. Look for high-quality  supplements that are free from contaminants.

## B Vitamins

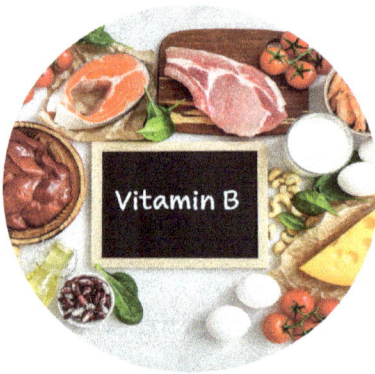

The B vitamins, particularly B6 (pyridoxine), B12 (cobalamin), and folate (B9), are crucial for brain health. These vitamins are involved in the synthesis of neurotransmitters such as serotonin, dopamine, and GABA, which regulate mood, cognition, and sleep. They also play a key role in the methylation process, which is critical for DNA repair, detoxification, and the production of brain chemicals.

Methylation is a critical biochemical process that affects gene expression, detoxification, and neurotransmitter production, all of which are essential for brain health. When methylation is impaired, often due to genetic mutations like MTHFR or environmental factors such as poor diet or toxin exposure, it can lead to a buildup of toxins and insufficient production of neurotransmitters like serotonin and dopamine.

This impairment is common, affecting at least 40% of the population. For individuals who are not effectively methylating, supplementing with methylated forms of B vitamins, such as methylfolate and methylcobalamin (B12), is crucial. These forms are more readily absorbed and utilized by the body, helping to support proper methylation, reduce neuroinflammation, and prevent brain issues like cognitive decline, mood disorders, and neurodevelopmental disorders.

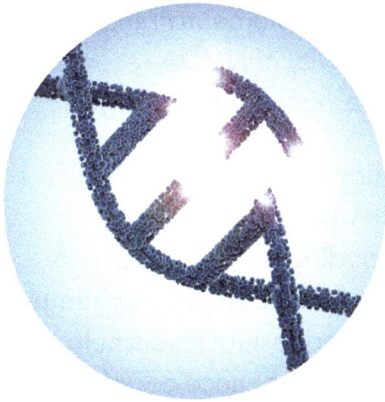

If someone is not properly methylating, they can accumulate a high level of homocysteine in the blood, which is linked to cognitive decline and an increased risk of neurodegenerative diseases, such as Alzheimer's and dementia, as it can lead to neuroinflammation, oxidative stress, and direct neurotoxicity. It is also associated with an increased risk of cardiovascular diseases, such as heart attack, stroke, and atherosclerosis, as it can damage the lining of blood vessels, promote blood clot formation, and contribute to arterial stiffness.

Adequate levels of B12 and folate are essential for preventing cognitive decline and maintaining mental clarity. B12 deficiency, in particular, is linked to memory loss, depression, and brain shrinkage. B6 supports the conversion of homocysteine, an amino acid that can be neurotoxic at high levels, into less harmful substances. Elevated homocysteine is associated with an increased risk of cognitive decline and Alzheimer's disease.

B6 is found in foods like poultry, fish, potatoes, and bananas. B12 is primarily found in animal products such as meat, fish, eggs, and dairy. Folate is abundant in leafy green vegetables, legumes, and fortified cereals. For those with dietary restrictions, B vitamin supplements, including methylated forms of B12 and folate, can help ensure adequate intake.

## Magnesium

Magnesium is a mineral that plays a pivotal role in brain health. It is involved in over 300 enzymatic reactions in the body, including those related to energy production, DNA synthesis, and neurotransmitter function. Magnesium also regulates the activity of NMDA receptors, which are critical for synaptic plasticity, memory, and learning.

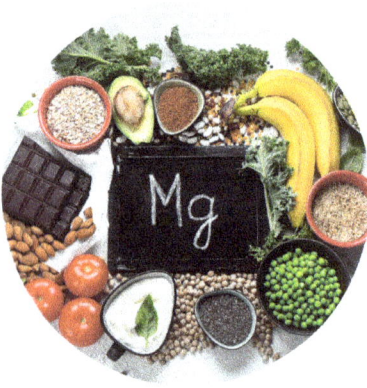

 Magnesium deficiency has been linked to a range of neurological issues, including migraines, anxiety, depression, and cognitive impairment. Adequate magnesium levels help to stabilize mood, enhance cognitive function, and protect against neurodegeneration. Magnesium also helps to regulate the body's stress response by modulating the release of cortisol, the stress hormone.

Magnesium-rich foods include leafy green vegetables (e.g., spinach, Swiss chard), nuts and seeds (e.g., almonds, pumpkin seeds), legumes, and whole grains.

There are different forms of magnesium in supplements, and they all target different functions. **Magnesium citrate** is great for bowels and constipation, **magnesium malate** targets muscle pain and improves energy levels, **magnesium glycinate** targets the nervous system, and

**magnesium L-Threonate** crosses the blood brain barrier the best, so is good for the brain.

## Antioxidants

Antioxidants play a crucial role in protecting the brain from oxidative stress, which occurs when free radicals (unstable molecules) damage cells and contribute to aging and disease. Vitamin C is a potent antioxidant that helps neutralize free radicals and supports the synthesis of neurotransmitters. Vitamin E, particularly in its natural form (alpha-tocopherol), protects cell membranes from oxidative damage and is essential for maintaining brain health.

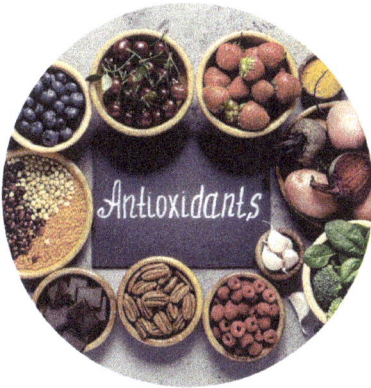

Antioxidants help to preserve cognitive function by reducing oxidative damage to brain cells. Studies have shown that higher levels of antioxidants in the diet are associated with a lower risk of cognitive decline and neurodegenerative diseases like Alzheimer's. Vitamin C is also involved in the production of collagen, which supports the structural integrity of blood vessels in the brain, ensuring adequate blood flow and nutrient delivery.

Citrus fruits, berries, bell peppers, and leafy greens are excellent sources of vitamin C. Vitamin E is found in nuts (e.g., almonds, hazelnuts), seeds, and vegetable oils (e.g., sunflower oil). Including a variety of colorful fruits and vegetables in your diet ensures a steady supply of antioxidants.

## Amino Acids

Amino acids are the building blocks of proteins and play a vital role in brain function. When protein is consumed, it should be completely digested to the amino acid state where it can be reconstructed by the body into new proteins.

One amino acid is tyrosine, a precursor to dopamine. It is a neurotransmitter that regulates mood, motivation, and focus. Tryptophan is a precursor to serotonin, the neurotransmitter that regulates mood, sleep, and appetite.

Adequate intake of these amino acids supports neurotransmitter production, enhancing mood, cognitive function, and stress resilience. Tyrosine has been shown to improve cognitive performance under stress, while tryptophan is known for its calming effects and ability to promote restful sleep.

Tyrosine is found in protein-rich foods like chicken, turkey, fish, dairy products, and nuts. Tryptophan is abundant in turkey, chicken, cheese, yogurt, and seeds. For those with specific needs, amino acid supplements can be used to support neurotransmitter balance. I particularly like MAP.

## Zinc

Zinc is an essential mineral involved in numerous aspects of cellular metabolism, including immune function, protein synthesis, and DNA repair. In the brain, zinc plays a critical role in synaptic transmission, neuroplasticity, and the regulation of neurotransmitters.

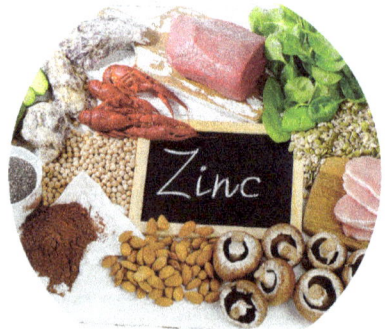

Zinc deficiency is associated with cognitive impairments, mood disorders, and neurodegenerative diseases. Zinc supports memory formation, learning, and overall cognitive function. It also has neuroprotective effects, helping to reduce inflammation and oxidative stress in the brain.

Zinc and copper balance each other and if one is up the other is down. Both zinc and copper are important for mental health, but it is common that people are copper toxic, resulting in anxiousness and the propensity to get sick. Pyroluria is a condition where zinc and B6 are bound and removed from the body, leaving the body deficient in both of these nutrients and an excess of zinc. This is common in people who have anxiety, especially social anxiety.

Zinc-rich foods include oysters, beef, poultry, beans, nuts, and whole grains. Zinc supplements, particularly in the form of zinc picolinate or zinc citrate, can help address deficiencies and support brain health.

## Iron

Iron is essential for the production of hemoglobin, the protein in red blood cells that carries oxygen to the brain and other tissues. Iron is also involved in the synthesis of neurotransmitters, including dopamine and serotonin, and supports overall brain function.

Iron deficiency, particularly in the form of anemia, can lead to fatigue, poor concentration, and cognitive decline. Adequate iron levels are necessary for maintaining energy levels, mental clarity, and cognitive performance.

Iron is found in both animal and plant-based foods. Heme iron, which is more easily absorbed by the body, is found in red meat, poultry, and fish. Non-heme iron is found in plant-based foods like lentils, beans, spinach, and fortified cereals. Consuming vitamin C-rich foods alongside iron-rich meals can enhance iron absorption.

## Vitamin D

Vitamin D is crucial for brain health, immune function, and mood regulation. If you have limited sun exposure or live in a region with long winters, a vitamin D supplement may be necessary to maintain optimal levels.

Vitamin D is best metabolized when taken with other cofactors, such as vitamin K2 and Vitamin A.  Therefore, it is optimal to take Vitamin D with a wide range of other nutrients.

Optimally you want your blood levels of Vitamin D to be 80 or above. Depending on your current levels, you will probably want to take around 5,000IU of Vitamin D daily.

## Phosphatidylserine & phosphatidylcholine

Phosphatidylserine is a phospholipid that supports cell membrane integrity and neurotransmitter function. It has been shown to improve memory, focus, and cognitive performance.

Phosphatidylcholine is a phospholipid and a major component of cell membranes, playing a crucial role in maintaining their structure and function. As a key building block of cell membranes, phosphatidylcholine helps maintain the fluidity and integrity of cells, supporting various cellular functions, including signal transmission, nutrient transport, and cell communication. In addition to its structural role, phosphatidylcholine is a precursor to acetylcholine, a neurotransmitter essential for memory, learning, and muscle control, making it important for brain health and cognitive function.

# Superfoods for Brain Health

In addition to ensuring you're getting the key nutrients your brain needs, certain superfoods can provide an extra boost to cognitive function. These foods are packed with nutrients and bioactive compounds that support brain health, improve memory, enhance focus, and protect against cognitive decline.

Here are some of the top superfoods for brain health:

## Blueberries

Blueberries are rich in antioxidants, particularly anthocyanins, which have been shown to protect the brain from oxidative stress and reduce inflammation. Blueberries also enhance communication between brain cells, improve memory, and support cognitive function.

Add fresh or frozen blueberries to smoothies, yogurt, oatmeal, or salads for a delicious and brain-boosting snack.

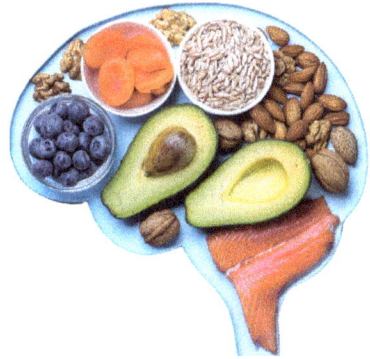

## Turmeric

Turmeric contains curcumin, a powerful anti-inflammatory and antioxidant compound that crosses the blood-brain barrier. Curcumin has been shown to enhance mood, improve memory, and protect against neurodegenerative diseases by reducing amyloid plaque buildup in the brain.

Use turmeric in cooking, add it to smoothies, or make a golden milk latte with turmeric, coconut milk, and a pinch of black pepper (which enhances curcumin absorption).

## Walnuts

Walnuts are rich in omega-3 fatty acids, antioxidants, and vitamin E, all of which support brain health. Regular consumption of walnuts has been associated with improved cognitive function, memory, and mood.

Enjoy walnuts as a snack, add them to salads, or use them in baking for a brain-boosting addition to your diet.

## Dark Chocolate

Dark chocolate, particularly varieties with 70% cocoa or higher (I personally prefer 85%), is rich in flavonoids, antioxidants that enhance blood flow to the brain and improve cognitive function. Dark chocolate also stimulates the production of endorphins and serotonin, which promote a positive mood.

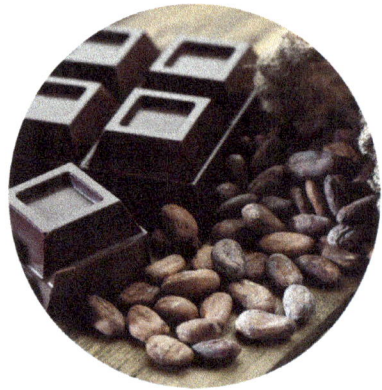

Enjoy a small piece of dark chocolate as a daily treat, add cocoa powder to smoothies, or use it in healthy baking recipes.

## Leafy Greens

Leafy greens like spinach, kale, and Swiss chard are packed with vitamins, minerals, and antioxidants that support brain health. They are rich in folate, vitamin K, and lutein, which protect the brain from oxidative damage and improve cognitive function.

Include leafy greens in salads, smoothies, stir-fries, and soups to boost your intake of brain-healthy nutrients.

## Avocado

Avocados are rich in healthy monounsaturated fats, which support blood flow to the brain and improve cognitive function. They are also a good source of vitamin E, an antioxidant that protects against oxidative stress.

Add avocado to salads, sandwiches, smoothies, or enjoy it as guacamole for a brain-boosting snack.

## Eggs

Eggs are an excellent source of choline, a nutrient that is essential for the production of acetylcholine, a neurotransmitter involved in memory and learning. Eggs also provide high-quality protein, B vitamins, and healthy fats that support brain health.

Enjoy eggs in a variety of ways—boiled, scrambled, poached, or as part of a veggie-packed omelet.

## Natural Nootropics for Brain Health

Nootropics, often referred to as "smart drugs" or cognitive enhancers, are substances that can enhance brain function, improve memory, increase focus, and boost overall cognitive performance. While synthetic nootropics are available, there is a growing interest in natural nootropics derived from herbs, plants, and other natural sources due to their safety profiles and additional health benefits.

Here are some of the most commonly used natural nootropics for brain health:

## 1. Bacopa Monnieri:

Bacopa Monnieri, also known as Brahmi, is an herb traditionally used in Ayurvedic medicine to enhance memory and cognitive function. It contains active compounds called bacosides, which have been shown to improve neuron communication and support brain function by promoting dendritic growth. Bacopa Monnieri is particularly beneficial for improving memory recall, reducing anxiety, and enhancing attention span. Studies have also suggested that it possesses antioxidant properties that protect brain cells from oxidative stress and age-related cognitive decline.

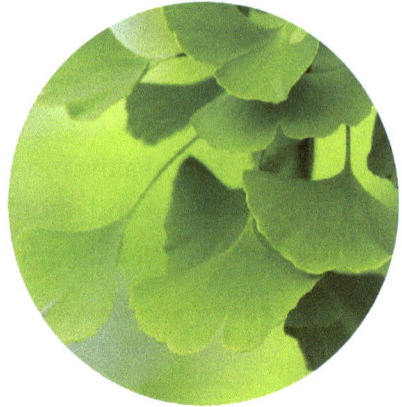

## 2. Ginkgo Biloba:

Ginkgo Biloba is one of the most widely used herbal supplements for cognitive enhancement. Extracted from the leaves of the Ginkgo tree, this nootropic is known for its ability to improve blood circulation to the brain, which can enhance oxygen and nutrient delivery to brain cells. This increased circulation can improve cognitive function, memory, and concentration. Ginkgo Biloba also has neuroprotective properties, helping to protect neurons from damage caused by free radicals. It has been particularly studied for its potential benefits in reducing symptoms of cognitive decline in older adults.

## 3. Rhodiola Rosea:

Rhodiola Rosea is an adaptogenic herb known for its ability to help the body adapt to stress and maintain mental clarity. It has been used traditionally in Russia and Scandinavian countries to combat fatigue and improve endurance. Rhodiola works by influencing key neurotransmitters, such as serotonin and dopamine, which are crucial for mood regulation and cognitive function. It can help reduce mental fatigue, enhance focus, and improve mood, making it particularly useful for individuals dealing with chronic stress or burnout.

### 4. Lion's Mane Mushroom:

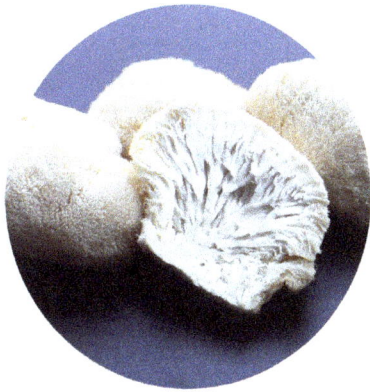

Lion's Mane is a unique type of mushroom with neuroprotective and neuroregenerative properties. It contains compounds called hericenones and erinacines, which can stimulate the production of nerve growth factor (NGF), a protein that supports the growth and maintenance of neurons. Lion's Mane is believed to enhance cognitive function, improve memory, and potentially support brain plasticity, making it beneficial for both short-term cognitive enhancement and long-term brain health. It is also being studied for its potential to slow the progression of neurodegenerative diseases like Alzheimer's.

### 5. Ashwagandha:

Ashwagandha is another adaptogenic herb with nootropic properties, widely used in traditional Ayurvedic medicine. It helps the body manage stress by modulating cortisol levels and supporting the adrenal glands. Ashwagandha has been shown to improve cognitive function, particularly in terms of reaction time, task performance, and memory. Its ability to reduce anxiety and stress while boosting overall mental clarity and concentration makes it an effective natural nootropic for enhancing brain function.

## 6. Panax Ginseng:

Panax Ginseng, also known as Asian Ginseng, is a well-known herbal remedy used to boost energy, reduce fatigue, and enhance cognitive function. Ginsenosides, the active compounds in Ginseng, are believed to improve mental performance by increasing acetylcholine levels in the brain, a neurotransmitter vital for learning and memory. Panax Ginseng has been studied for its potential to improve cognitive performance, mental energy, and focus, particularly in people experiencing mental fatigue or cognitive decline.

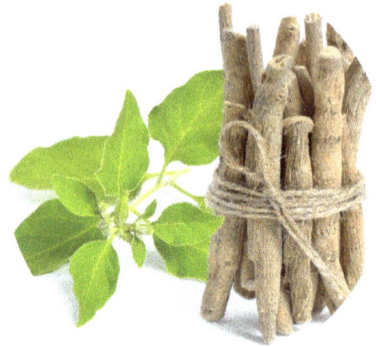

## 7. L-Theanine:

L-Theanine is an amino acid found primarily in green tea leaves. It is known for its relaxing effects without causing drowsiness, making it an ideal nootropic for enhancing mental clarity and focus. L-Theanine promotes the production of alpha brain waves, which are associated with a relaxed yet alert mental state. It can also increase levels of neurotransmitters like serotonin and dopamine, which help improve mood and cognitive function. L-Theanine is often used in combination with caffeine to provide a balanced boost in focus and alertness without the jittery side effects commonly associated with caffeine.

## 8. Curcumin:

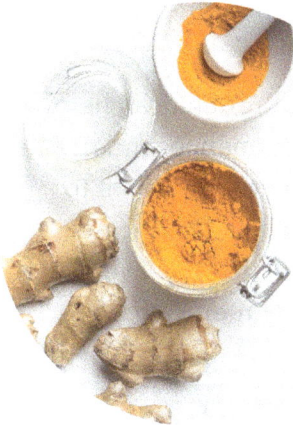

Curcumin is the active compound found in turmeric, a spice widely used in cooking and traditional medicine. It has potent anti-inflammatory and antioxidant properties, which help protect the brain from damage caused by oxidative stress and inflammation. Curcumin can cross the blood-brain barrier and has been shown to increase levels of brain-derived neurotrophic factor (BDNF), a protein that supports the growth and survival of neurons. Studies suggest that curcumin may help improve memory, reduce symptoms of depression, and protect against cognitive decline associated with aging and neurodegenerative diseases.

## 9. Gotu Kola:

Gotu Kola is an herb used in traditional Chinese and Ayurvedic medicine for its cognitive-enhancing and neuroprotective properties. It is believed to improve memory, reduce anxiety, and enhance overall cognitive function by supporting the health of blood vessels and improving circulation, including within the brain. Gotu Kola also has adaptogenic properties, helping to reduce the effects of stress on the body and mind, which can improve focus and mental clarity.

## 10. Huperzine A:

Huperzine A is a compound extracted from the Chinese club moss plant. It is known for its ability to inhibit acetylcholinesterase, an enzyme that breaks down acetylcholine, a neurotransmitter essential for learning and memory. By preventing the breakdown of acetylcholine, Huperzine A can enhance cognitive function, improve memory retention, and increase alertness. It is often used as a natural nootropic to support cognitive performance and has been studied for its potential benefits in managing symptoms of Alzheimer's disease.

Incorporating these natural nootropics into your routine can help enhance brain function, improve cognitive performance, and protect against age-related cognitive decline. However, it's important to choose high-quality supplements and consult with a healthcare professional before starting any new regimen, especially if you have pre-existing health conditions or are taking other medications.

# Conclusion: Building a Brain-Healthy Diet

Nourishing your brain is one of the most powerful steps you can take to optimize cognitive function, enhance mood, and protect against cognitive decline. By prioritizing a diet rich in brain-healthy nutrients, supporting gut health, incorporating superfoods, and considering targeted supplementation, you can fuel your brain for peak performance and longevity.

Remember, the foundation of brain health begins with the choices you make every day. By making thoughtful decisions about what you eat, how you live, and how you care for your body, you can create an environment in which your brain can thrive.

In the next chapter, we'll explore the fourth step in the 5-step model: balancing the nervous system. Once your brain is well-nourished, it's essential to ensure that your nervous system is in a state of balance, allowing you to manage stress effectively, stay calm under pressure, and maintain emotional stability.

# 5

# Step 4
# – Balancing the Nervous System

## Introduction: The Foundation of Emotional and Cognitive Stability

The nervous system is the body's command center, responsible for processing information, regulating bodily functions, and coordinating the brain's response to stimuli. It's divided into two main parts: the central nervous system (CNS), which includes the brain and spinal cord, and the peripheral nervous system (PNS), which connects the CNS to the rest of the body. Within the PNS, the autonomic nervous system (ANS) plays a critical role in regulating involuntary bodily functions, such as heart rate, digestion, and respiratory rate.

The autonomic nervous system is further divided into two branches: the sympathetic nervous system (SNS), which triggers the "fight or flight" response, and the parasympathetic nervous system (PNS), which promotes "rest and digest" activities. A balanced nervous system allows the body to switch smoothly between these states, ensuring that you can handle stress effectively, maintain emotional stability, and support cognitive function.

However, in today's fast-paced world, many people find themselves stuck in a state of sympathetic dominance, where the "fight or flight" response is constantly activated. This chronic stress state can lead to a host of issues, including anxiety, insomnia, digestive problems, and cognitive dysfunction. Balancing the nervous system is essential for restoring emotional and cognitive stability, enhancing resilience to stress, and supporting overall well-being.

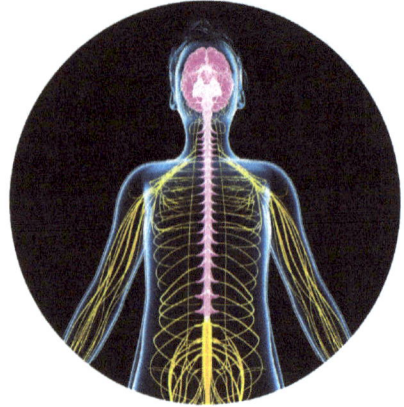

In this chapter, we'll explore the importance of nervous system balance, the impact of chronic stress on brain health, and practical strategies for calming the nervous system and promoting a state of balance and relaxation.

## Understanding the Autonomic Nervous System

The autonomic nervous system (ANS) operates largely below the level of consciousness, controlling involuntary functions such as heart rate, blood pressure, digestion, and respiratory rate. It's responsible for maintaining homeostasis, or the body's internal balance, by regulating these processes in response to internal and external stimuli.

The ANS is divided into two main branches:

## 1. The Sympathetic Nervous System (SNS):

The SNS is responsible for the body's "fight or flight" response. When you perceive a threat–whether physical, emotional, or psychological– the SNS is activated, preparing the body to either confront or flee from the danger. This response involves increasing heart rate, dilating pupils, slowing digestion, and releasing stress hormones like cortisol and adrenaline.

While the "fight or flight" response is essential for survival, chronic activation of the SNS can have detrimental effects on brain health. Prolonged exposure to stress hormones can damage brain cells, particularly in areas like the hippocampus (responsible for memory) and the prefrontal cortex (responsible for decision-making and emotional regulation). Chronic stress can also lead to anxiety, depression, and cognitive decline.

## 2. The Parasympathetic Nervous System (PNS):

The PNS is often referred to as the "rest and digest" system. It promotes relaxation, recovery, and healing by slowing the heart rate, stimulating digestion, and conserving energy. The PNS is activated during times of rest, allowing the body to repair and regenerate.

Activation of the PNS supports brain health by reducing inflammation, promoting neurogenesis (the formation of new neurons), and enhancing cognitive function. A well-functioning PNS helps maintain emotional stability, supports healthy sleep, and improves resilience to stress.

For optimal brain health and well-being, it's crucial to maintain a balance between these two branches of the ANS. However, in modern society, many people experience chronic stress, leading to a state of sympathetic dominance, where the SNS is overactive, and the PNS is underactive.

# The Impact of Chronic Stress on the Nervous System

Chronic stress is one of the most significant factors that disrupt the balance of the autonomic nervous system. When the body is exposed to prolonged stress—whether from work pressure, financial concerns, relationship issues, or health problems—the SNS remains activated, leading to an overproduction of stress hormones like cortisol and adrenaline. Over time, this can have a profound impact on both physical and mental health.

Here's how chronic stress affects the nervous system and brain health:

## Increased Cortisol Levels:

Cortisol, the primary stress hormone, plays a key role in the body's response to stress. However, when cortisol levels remain elevated for extended periods, it can lead to neurotoxicity and damage to brain cells. High cortisol levels have been associated with shrinkage of the hippocampus, leading to memory problems and impaired learning. Cortisol also affects the prefrontal cortex, reducing cognitive function and emotional regulation.

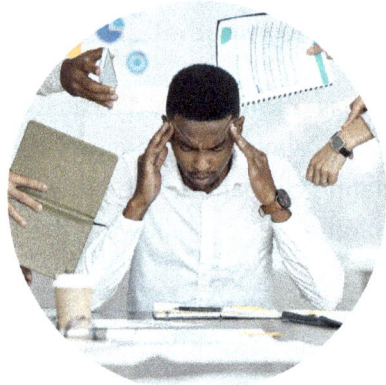

Chronic stress and elevated cortisol levels suppress the immune system, making the body more susceptible to infections and illnesses. This can lead to a cycle of poor health and further stress, exacerbating the imbalance of the nervous system.

## Sympathetic Dominance:

Sympathetic dominance is characterized by a heightened state of arousal and vigilance, even in the absence of immediate threats. This state can lead to physical symptoms such as increased heart rate, high blood pressure, muscle tension, and digestive issues. Over time, sympathetic dominance can contribute to the development of chronic conditions such as hypertension, heart disease, and gastrointestinal disorders.

Sympathetic dominance is also associated with mental health issues such as anxiety, panic attacks, and insomnia. The constant activation of the "fight or flight" response can lead to hypervigilance, irritability, and difficulty relaxing, all of which contribute to a decline in mental well-being.

## Reduced Neuroplasticity:

Neuroplasticity refers to the brain's ability to reorganize itself by forming new neural connections. Chronic stress can reduce neuroplasticity, making it harder for the brain to adapt, learn, and recover from injury. This can lead to cognitive decline, difficulty learning new information, and impaired problem-solving skills.

Reduced neuroplasticity also affects the brain's ability to regulate emotions. Individuals with chronic stress may experience mood swings, depression, and difficulty coping with emotional challenges.

## Disrupted Sleep Patterns:

Sleep is essential for brain health, as it allows the brain to repair itself, consolidate memories, and clear out toxins. Chronic stress can disrupt sleep patterns, leading to insomnia, restless sleep, and difficulty falling or staying asleep. Poor sleep quality further exacerbates stress, creating a vicious cycle that impairs cognitive function and emotional well-being.

Disrupted sleep patterns can also affect physical health, leading to fatigue, weakened immune function, and increased risk of chronic diseases such as diabetes and obesity.

# Strategies for Balancing the Nervous System

Balancing the nervous system requires a multifaceted approach that addresses both the physical and psychological aspects of stress. By implementing strategies to activate the parasympathetic nervous system and reduce sympathetic dominance, you can restore balance to the nervous system, enhance brain health, and improve overall well-being.

Here are some effective strategies for balancing the nervous system:

## Mindfulness and Meditation

Mindfulness and meditation are powerful tools for activating the parasympathetic nervous system and reducing the effects of chronic stress. These practices involve focusing on the present moment, cultivating awareness, and letting go of negative thoughts and emotions. Regular meditation has been shown to reduce cortisol levels, improve emotional regulation, and enhance neuroplasticity.

Start with short, daily meditation sessions, gradually increasing the duration as you become more comfortable with the practice. There are various forms of meditation to explore, including mindfulness meditation, loving-kindness meditation, and guided visualization. Apps and online resources can provide guided meditations and help you establish a consistent practice. Joe Dispenza is a great resource and a great place to start. He has a lot of free online guided meditations.

## Breathwork

Breathwork involves conscious control of breathing patterns to influence the nervous system. Deep, slow breathing activates the parasympathetic nervous system, promoting relaxation and reducing the "fight or flight" response. Breathwork can also improve oxygen delivery to the brain, enhancing cognitive function and mental clarity.

Practice deep breathing exercises, such as diaphragmatic breathing, box breathing, or the 4-7-8 technique. Diaphragmatic breathing involves breathing deeply into the abdomen, rather than shallowly into the chest. Box breathing involves inhaling for four counts, holding the breath for four counts, exhaling for four counts, and holding again for four counts. The 4-7-8 technique involves inhaling for four counts, holding for seven counts, and exhaling for eight counts. Incorporate breathwork into your daily routine, especially during times of stress or anxiety.

## Yoga and Tai Chi

Yoga and Tai Chi are mind-body practices that combine physical movement, breath control, and meditation to promote balance in the nervous system. These practices enhance flexibility, strength, and body awareness while also reducing stress and anxiety. Yoga, in particular, has been shown to reduce cortisol levels, improve mood, and enhance cognitive function.

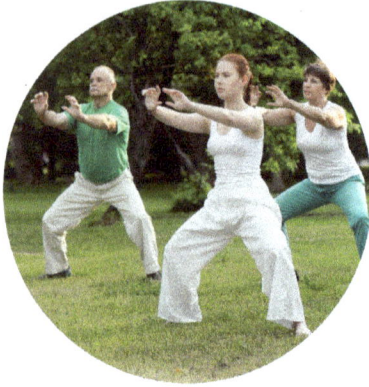

Incorporate yoga or Tai Chi into your regular exercise routine. Many styles of yoga, such as Hatha, Vinyasa, and Yin yoga, focus on different aspects of physical and mental well-being. Tai Chi, a Chinese martial art, emphasizes slow, deliberate movements and deep breathing. Both practices can be done in a group setting, at home with online classes, or as part of a personal daily routine.

## Vagus Nerve Stimulation

The vagus nerve is the longest cranial nerve and plays a crucial role in regulating the parasympathetic nervous system. Stimulating the vagus nerve can promote relaxation, reduce inflammation, and enhance mood. The vagus nerve runs down by the throat, so activities that involve the throat area stimulate the vagus nerve include deep breathing, singing, humming, and cold exposure.

 Practice vagus nerve stimulation techniques regularly to activate the parasympathetic nervous system. For example, singing or humming for a few minutes each day can stimulate the vagus nerve and promote relaxation. Cold exposure, such as taking cold showers or applying cold packs to the face, can also stimulate the vagus nerve and reduce stress.

## Physical Activity

Regular physical activity is essential for maintaining a balanced nervous system. Exercise helps regulate stress hormones, improve mood, and enhance cognitive function. It also promotes better sleep, which is crucial for nervous system recovery and overall brain health. Physical activity stimulates the production of endorphins, neurotransmitters that act as natural mood enhancers.

Engage in regular aerobic exercise, such as walking, running, swimming, or cycling, for at least 150 minutes per week. Strength training exercises, such as weightlifting or bodyweight exercises, should also be incorporated into your routine to build muscle and improve physical resilience. Additionally, practices like yoga or Tai Chi can be included to enhance flexibility, balance, and mental well-being.

## Healthy Sleep Habits

Sleep is vital for nervous system balance, as it allows the body to recover from daily stressors and the brain to consolidate memories and clear out toxins. Prioritizing sleep and establishing healthy sleep habits can reduce sympathetic dominance and support overall brain health.

Aim for 7-9 hours of quality sleep each night. Establish a consistent sleep schedule by going to bed and waking up at the same time each day, even on weekends. Create a sleep-friendly environment by keeping your bedroom cool, dark, and quiet. Limit exposure to screens before bed, as the blue light emitted by devices can disrupt melatonin production. Consider using relaxation techniques, such as meditation or deep breathing, to wind down before bedtime.

**Nutrition for Nervous System Balance**

Nutrition plays a crucial role in supporting nervous system balance and brain health. Certain nutrients, such as omega-3 fatty acids, magnesium, and B vitamins, help regulate neurotransmitter function, reduce inflammation, and support stress resilience.

Incorporate a variety of nutrient-dense foods into your diet, including fatty fish (rich in omega-3s), leafy greens (high in magnesium and B vitamins), nuts and seeds, and whole grains. Avoid excessive consumption of caffeine, sugar, and processed foods, which can exacerbate stress and contribute to nervous system imbalance. Consider taking supplements, such as magnesium or B-complex vitamins, if you're not getting enough of these nutrients through your diet.

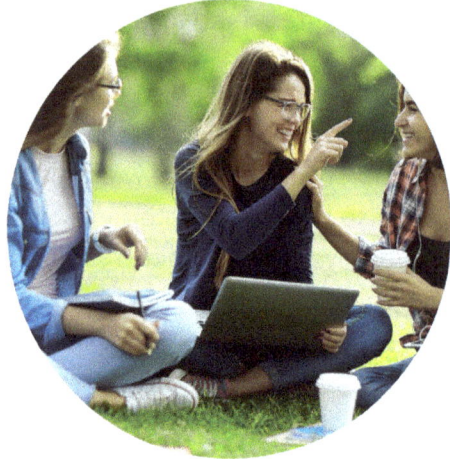

# Social Connections and Emotional Support

Social connections and emotional support are vital for mental health and nervous system balance. Positive social interactions reduce stress, enhance mood, and provide a sense of belonging and purpose. Having a strong support network can help you cope with life's challenges and reduce the impact of stress on the nervous system.

Cultivate meaningful relationships with family, friends, and community members. Make time for regular social activities, whether in person or virtually, to strengthen your support network. Engage in open and honest communication with loved ones, and seek support when needed. If you're feeling isolated, consider joining clubs, groups, or organizations that align with your interests and values.

## Limiting Exposure to Stressors

Reducing exposure to unnecessary stressors can help prevent sympathetic dominance and support nervous system balance. By identifying and managing sources of stress in your life, you can create a more peaceful and supportive environment for your mental and physical well-being.

Assess your daily life for sources of stress, such as a demanding work environment, toxic relationships, or unhealthy habits. Take proactive steps to reduce or eliminate these stressors. This may involve setting boundaries at work, seeking therapy or counseling, or making lifestyle changes to prioritize self-care. Practice time management and organization to reduce overwhelm and create a sense of control over your responsibilities.

# Advanced Techniques for Nervous System Regulation

For individuals who experience significant stress or have difficulty balancing their nervous system through conventional methods, advanced techniques may provide additional support. These techniques can be used in conjunction with the strategies mentioned above to enhance nervous system balance and improve brain health.

# Biofeedback

Biofeedback is a therapeutic technique that involves using electronic monitoring devices to measure physiological functions, such as heart rate, muscle tension, and brainwave activity. By providing real-time feedback, biofeedback allows individuals to gain greater awareness of their physiological responses and learn how to control them. Biofeedback has been shown to reduce stress, anxiety, and symptoms of PTSD.

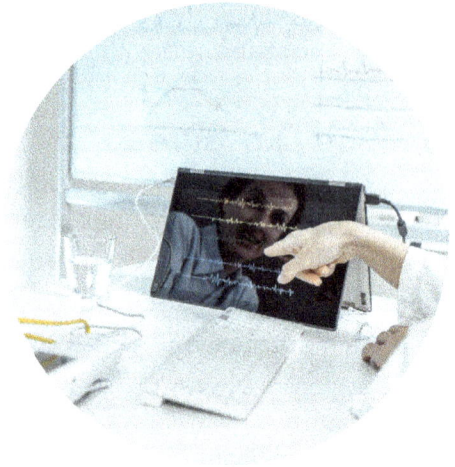

Biofeedback therapy is typically conducted by a trained therapist using specialized equipment. However, there are also home-based biofeedback devices available that allow individuals to practice self-regulation techniques independently. Biofeedback sessions typically involve relaxation exercises, guided imagery, or mindfulness practices.

# Heart Rate Variability (HRV) Training

Heart rate variability (HRV) refers to the variation in time between heartbeats, which is regulated by the autonomic nervous system. Higher HRV is associated with greater resilience to stress and better overall health. HRV training involves using biofeedback to monitor HRV and practice techniques to improve it, such as deep breathing, meditation, and physical exercise.

HRV training can be done using biofeedback devices that monitor heart rate and provide feedback on HRV. By practicing techniques that promote relaxation and balance, individuals can improve their HRV and enhance nervous system regulation.

## Neurofeedback

Neurofeedback, also known as EEG biofeedback, is a form of biofeedback that involves monitoring brainwave activity and providing real-time feedback to help individuals regulate their brain function. Neurofeedback can be used to treat a variety of conditions, including anxiety, depression, ADHD, and PTSD. By training the brain to achieve a more balanced state, neurofeedback can improve cognitive function, emotional regulation, and stress resilience.

Neurofeedback is typically conducted by a trained therapist using specialized equipment that monitors brainwave activity. During a neurofeedback session, the individual receives visual or auditory feedback that reflects their brainwave patterns. Through repeated sessions, individuals learn to regulate their brainwave activity and achieve a more balanced state.

# Conclusion: Achieving Nervous System Balance for Optimal Brain Health

Balancing the nervous system is essential for maintaining emotional and cognitive stability, enhancing resilience to stress, and supporting overall brain health. By implementing a combination of mindfulness practices, breathwork, physical activity, healthy sleep habits, and advanced techniques like biofeedback and neurofeedback, you can restore balance to your autonomic nervous system and promote a state of relaxation and well-being.

Remember that achieving nervous system balance is an ongoing process that requires consistency and commitment. By making these practices a regular part of your life, you can create a strong foundation for long-term brain health, emotional stability, and cognitive resilience.

In the next chapter, we'll explore the final step in the 5-step model: rewiring the brain. Once your nervous system is balanced, you can focus on enhancing neuroplasticity and building new neural connections to improve cognitive function, memory, and mental agility

# 6

## Step 5
## – Rewiring the Brain

### Introduction: The Power of Neuroplasticity

Neuroplasticity is one of the most remarkable aspects of the human brain. It refers to the brain's ability to reorganize itself by forming new neural connections throughout life. This capability allows the brain to adapt to new experiences, learn new information, and recover from injury. The concept of neuroplasticity is central to the idea that you can "rewire" your brain to improve cognitive function, enhance memory, and increase mental agility.

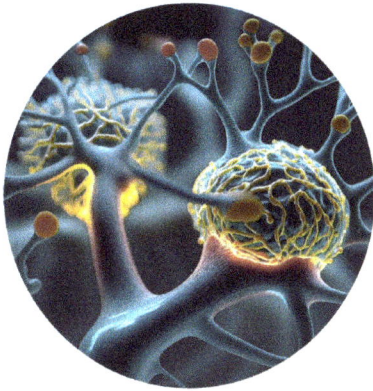

Rewiring the brain is not about making a few superficial changes; it's about creating lasting transformations in how your brain operates. Whether you want to overcome cognitive challenges, enhance your mental performance, or achieve greater emotional resilience, harnessing the power of neuroplasticity can lead to significant improvements in your brain's capabilities.

In this chapter, we'll explore the science of neuroplasticity, practical strategies for rewiring the brain, and how to create an environment that supports ongoing brain development and optimization. Additionally, we'll delve into brain training techniques, the importance of stimulating the frontal lobe, and how tools like the Interactive Metronome can play a crucial role in enhancing brain function.

## The Science of Neuroplasticity

For many years, scientists believed that the adult brain was relatively fixed and unchangeable, with a limited capacity for growth and adaptation. However, research over the past few decades has revealed that the brain is far more dynamic and adaptable than previously thought. Neuroplasticity allows the brain to change its structure and function in response to learning, experience, and even injury.

Synaptic plasticity refers to the ability of synapses—the connections between neurons—to strengthen or weaken over time in response to activity levels. When you repeatedly engage in a particular thought or behavior, the synapses involved in that activity become stronger and more efficient. Conversely, synapses that are rarely used may weaken and eventually disappear.

Synaptic plasticity is the foundation of learning and memory. When you learn a new skill, such as playing a musical instrument or speaking a new language, your brain creates and strengthens synapses that support that skill. Over time, these connections become more efficient, allowing you to perform the skill with greater ease and accuracy.

Neurogenesis is the process of generating new neurons in the brain. For many years, it was believed that neurogenesis only occurred during early development, but research has shown that the adult brain can also produce new neurons, particularly in the hippocampus, an area critical for memory and learning.

Neurogenesis plays a crucial role in maintaining cognitive function, mood regulation, and emotional resilience. By promoting neurogenesis, you can enhance your brain's capacity for learning, improve memory, and reduce the risk of neurodegenerative diseases.

Understanding these mechanisms of neuroplasticity is essential for implementing strategies that support brain rewiring. By actively engaging in practices that promote neuroplasticity, you can enhance your brain's capacity to adapt, learn, and thrive.

# The Role of the Frontal Lobe in Brain Rewiring

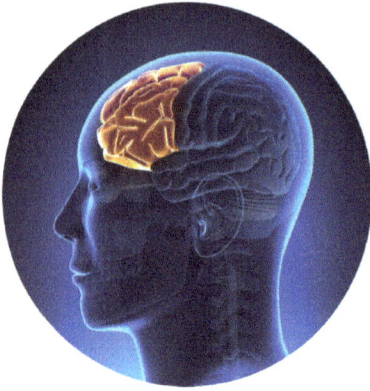

The frontal lobe plays a pivotal role in higher cognitive functions, such as decision-making, problem-solving, and emotional regulation. It's also deeply involved in executive functions like planning, impulse control, and attention. Given its central role in these functions, stimulating the frontal lobe is crucial for effective brain rewiring.

One of the most fascinating aspects of the frontal lobe is its inverse relationship with the amygdala, the brain's center for emotional responses, including fear and anxiety. When the frontal lobe is actively engaged in tasks that require focus, planning, or logical reasoning, it helps down-regulate the amygdala, thereby reducing emotional reactivity and promoting a state of calm and rational thinking.

## Stimulating the Frontal Lobe to Down-Regulate the Amygdala

The amygdala is responsible for the brain's "fight or flight" response, which can be triggered by stress, anxiety, or fear. While this response is crucial for survival, chronic activation of the amygdala can lead to heightened anxiety, stress, and emotional dysregulation. By engaging in activities that stimulate the frontal lobe, you can help balance the brain's emotional and cognitive responses, leading to improved mental clarity, emotional stability, and decision-making.

## How to Stimulate the Frontal Lobe:

Engaging in activities that challenge your executive functions can stimulate the frontal lobe. Examples include problem-solving tasks, strategy games like chess, complex puzzles, and tasks that require planning and organization.

Practices that require focused attention, such as mindfulness meditation, can activate the frontal lobe while calming the amygdala. Regular meditation has been shown to increase the thickness of the prefrontal cortex, enhancing its ability to regulate emotions and reduce stress.

Creative activities that involve planning, decision-making, and problem-solving, such as writing, drawing, or composing music, engage the frontal lobe and promote neuroplasticity.

By regularly engaging in these types of activities, you can strengthen the connections within the frontal lobe, leading to better emotional regulation, reduced anxiety, and enhanced cognitive function.

# Brain Training: A Key to Rewiring the Brain

Brain training involves structured exercises that target specific cognitive functions to improve memory, attention, problem-solving skills, and overall mental performance. The goal of brain training is to enhance neuroplasticity by challenging the brain in ways that promote the formation of new neural connections.

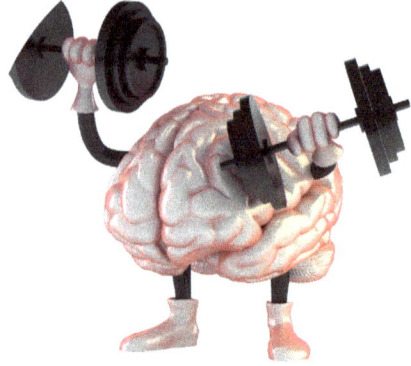

## The Importance of Brain Training

Just like physical exercise strengthens muscles, brain training strengthens cognitive functions. By regularly challenging your brain with targeted exercises, you can improve mental agility, enhance memory, and increase your brain's resilience to aging and stress.

Brain training typically targets key cognitive areas, such as memory, attention, processing speed, and executive function. By focusing on these areas, you can improve your overall cognitive performance and support long-term brain health.

Brain training promotes neuroplasticity by providing consistent cognitive challenges that encourage the brain to form new connections and strengthen existing ones. This process not only improves cognitive function but also supports emotional regulation and stress resilience.

Regular brain training has been shown to protect against age-related cognitive decline and reduce the risk of neurodegenerative diseases.

By keeping your brain active and engaged, you can maintain mental sharpness and adaptability throughout your life.

## Types of Brain Training Exercises

**Memory Exercises:** These exercises are designed to improve your ability to store and recall information. Examples include memory games, such as matching pairs, recalling sequences, or memorizing lists of words or numbers.

**Attention and Focus Exercises:** These exercises enhance your ability to concentrate and maintain focus on tasks. Examples include tasks that require sustained attention, such as tracking moving objects, filtering out distractions, or completing complex sequences.

**Problem-Solving and Logic Exercises:** These exercises challenge your critical thinking and problem-solving abilities. Examples include logic puzzles, strategy games, and tasks that require you to analyze information and make decisions based on that analysis.

**Multitasking Exercises:** Multitasking exercises improve your ability to manage multiple tasks simultaneously, enhancing cognitive flexibility and processing speed. Examples include games that require you to switch between different tasks quickly or manage several tasks at once..

## Neurofeedback

Besides helping with anxiety and regulating the nervous system, neurofeedback is also great for creating new neural networks. Usually neurofeed needs to be done with a professional, however, today there are several at home devices that are quite good.  My favorite system is Vital Neuro®.

# The Vital Neuro®: A Powerful At-Home Neurofeedback device

The **Vital Neuro Device** is a cutting-edge neurotechnology tool designed to enhance brain function through personalized brainwave entrainment and neurofeedback. The device leverages real-time EEG (electroencephalogram) monitoring to analyze the user's brainwave patterns and then uses specific audio and visual stimuli to guide the brain into optimal states of relaxation, focus, or cognitive performance. This process, known as brainwave entrainment, encourages the brain to synchronize its electrical activity to the desired frequency range, such as alpha (relaxed), beta (focused), or theta (meditative) brainwaves.

## How It Works:

The Vital Neuro Device operates by detecting the brain's electrical activity through sensors that are typically embedded in a wearable headset. Once the device gathers brainwave data, it processes this information to determine the current mental state of the user. Based on this real-time analysis, the device generates customized auditory and visual stimuli—often in the form of soundscapes, music, or light patterns—that are specifically designed to encourage the brain to shift towards a more desirable state. For example, if the device detects high levels of stress-related beta waves, it may produce calming alpha wave-inducing sounds to

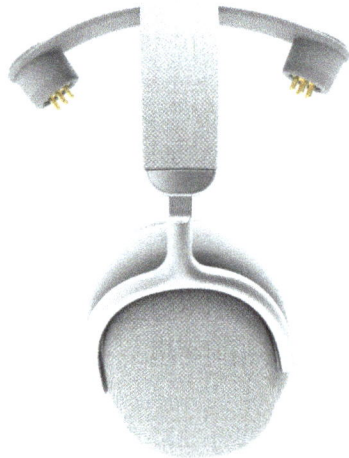

promote relaxation and stress reduction. The continuous feedback loop helps the brain learn to maintain or return to these beneficial states more easily over time.

## Benefits:

**Improved Cognitive Performance:** By training the brain to achieve optimal brainwave states, the Vital Neuro Device can enhance cognitive functions such as attention, memory, and problem-solving. Users often report sharper focus, quicker thinking, and improved learning capabilities.

**Stress Reduction and Relaxation:** The device can help users manage stress and anxiety by promoting relaxation and reducing excessive beta wave activity associated with stress. This makes it a valuable tool for stress management and mental wellness.

**Enhanced Sleep Quality:** By guiding the brain into deep relaxation and meditative states, the Vital Neuro Device can improve sleep onset and quality, helping users achieve more restful and restorative sleep.

**Support for Mental Health:** The device is useful in supporting mental health management, particularly for conditions like anxiety, depression, and ADHD, where brainwave imbalances are often present. It provides a non-invasive, drug-free approach to improving mental well-being.

**Peak Performance Training:** Athletes, executives, and performers use the Vital Neuro Device to enter a "flow state," a highly productive mental state characterized by deep focus and reduced internal distractions. This helps enhance performance in competitive or high-pressure situations.

## Applications:

The Vital Neuro Device is versatile and can be used across various settings and applications, including:

**Clinical and Therapeutic Settings:** Mental health professionals and neurofeedback therapists use the device to help patients with anxiety, depression, ADHD, PTSD, and other neurological conditions by training their brains towards healthier patterns.

**Home Use for Wellness and Relaxation:** Individuals use the device at home to enhance relaxation, manage stress, and improve sleep quality as part of a daily wellness routine.

**Corporate Wellness Programs:** Companies incorporate the Vital Neuro Device into corporate wellness programs to reduce employee stress, enhance focus, and boost productivity.

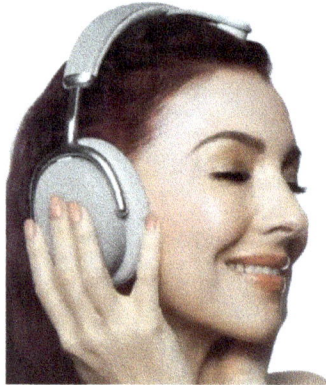

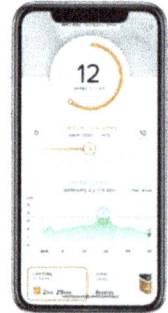

**Athletic and Performance Training:** Athletes and performers use the device to improve mental resilience, concentration, and the ability to enter and maintain a peak performance state.

The Vital Neuro Device represents a blend of modern neuroscience and technology, offering a practical tool for enhancing brain health and cognitive performance through targeted neurofeedback and brainwave entrainment. By training the brain to operate in optimal states, users can experience significant improvements in mental clarity, emotional balance, and overall cognitive function.

If you are interested in this device, I have placed a link at the end of this book so you can learn more. However, please contact me so that I may assist you in placing an order, as I will receive a modest commission.

# The Interactive Metronome®: A Powerful Tool for Brain Rewiring

The Interactive Metronome® (IM) is an advanced brain training tool that combines the principles of neuroplasticity with the precision of metronome-based timing exercises. It's designed to improve cognitive and motor function by training the brain to process information more efficiently.

## How the Interactive Metronome® Works

The IM involves performing specific movements, such as clapping hands or tapping feet, in time with a metronome beat. The device measures the accuracy of these movements, providing immediate feedback on how closely your actions align with the beat.

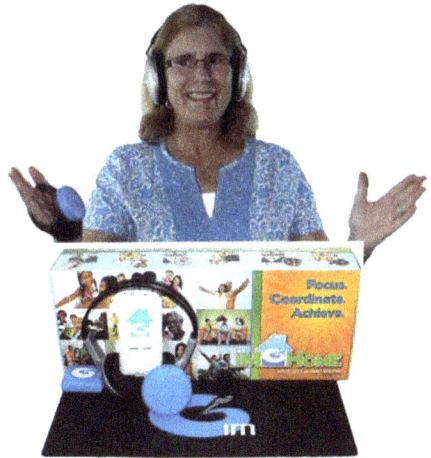

The IM provides visual and auditory feedback that helps you adjust your timing to match the metronome more accurately. This real-time feedback encourages the brain to fine-tune its processing and coordination, leading to improved cognitive and motor skills.

### 1. Benefits of the Interactive Metronome

The IM is particularly effective for improving attention, focus, and processing speed. By training the brain to synchronize movements with precise timing, the IM enhances the brain's ability to process information quickly and accurately.

: In addition to cognitive benefits, the IM also improves motor coordination and timing. This is particularly beneficial for individuals with motor coordination challenges, such as those with ADHD or developmental disorders.

The IM engages the frontal lobe by requiring sustained attention, precise timing, and decision-making. This engagement helps strengthen the neural connections in the frontal lobe, supporting emotional regulation and reducing the overactivity of the amygdala.

### 2. Applications of the Interactive Metronome

The IM is widely used in rehabilitation settings for individuals recovering from brain injuries, strokes, or developmental disorders. It helps improve cognitive and motor function, supporting the recovery process.

The IM is also used by students and professionals to enhance focus, attention, and cognitive performance. By improving timing and processing speed, the IM can lead to better academic and work outcomes.

Athletes use the IM to improve timing, coordination, and reaction speed. The precision required by the IM helps athletes refine their skills and perform at their best in high-pressure situations.

If you are interested in this device, I have placed a link at the end of this book so you can learn more. However, you need a practitioner in order to run this program from home. Please contact me so that I may assist you in setting up your account.

# Practical Strategies for Rewiring the Brain

Rewiring the brain involves engaging in activities and practices that promote the formation of new neural connections and strengthen existing ones. By incorporating these strategies into your daily life, you can enhance your brain's adaptability, improve cognitive function, and achieve greater mental resilience.

### 1. Engage in Lifelong Learning

Lifelong learning is one of the most effective ways to promote neuroplasticity. The brain thrives on new information and challenges, and learning provides the stimulus needed to create and strengthen neural connections.

Continuously seek out opportunities for learning and intellectual growth. This could involve formal education, such as taking classes or earning certifications, or informal learning, such as reading books, watching documentaries, or exploring new hobbies. The key is to keep your brain engaged with new and diverse experiences.

### 2. Practice Mindfulness and Meditation

Mindfulness and meditation have been shown to enhance neuroplasticity by improving attention, emotional regulation, and self-awareness. These practices encourage the brain to form new connections and break free from habitual thought patterns.

Incorporate mindfulness practices into your daily routine, such as mindful breathing, body scanning, or mindful eating. Set aside time each day for meditation, starting with short sessions and gradually increasing the duration as you become more comfortable. Use apps or guided meditations to help you establish a consistent practice.

### 3. Challenge Your Brain with Puzzles and Games

Puzzles and brain games stimulate cognitive function by challenging your memory, problem-solving skills, and critical thinking. These activities engage multiple areas of the brain, promoting neuroplasticity and improving mental agility.

Dedicate time each day to engaging in puzzles and brain games, such as crosswords, Sudoku, chess, or memory games. Consider trying online brain training programs that offer a variety of cognitive challenges tailored to your skill level. Vary the types of puzzles and games you play to ensure that your brain is continually exposed to new and different challenges.

### 4. Explore Creative Activities

Creativity involves thinking outside the box, exploring new ideas, and experimenting with different approaches. Creative activities engage the brain in unique ways, encouraging the formation of new neural connections and enhancing cognitive flexibility.

Explore creative activities that interest you, such as painting, writing, music, photography, or crafting. Allow yourself to experiment and take risks without worrying about the outcome. Creative expression can also be a powerful way to process emotions, reduce stress, and improve overall well-being.

### 5. Incorporate Multisensory Learning

Multisensory learning involves engaging multiple senses simultaneously, which enhances memory retention and cognitive function. When you learn through sight, sound, touch, and movement, your brain creates stronger and more diverse neural connections.

Incorporate multisensory techniques into your learning experiences. For example, if you're learning a new language, listen to audio recordings, watch videos, and practice speaking aloud while writing down new vocabulary. In hands-on activities, such as cooking or gardening, pay attention to the sights, sounds, smells, and textures involved. Multisensory learning can also be applied to studying, teaching, or presenting information.

### 6. Use Visualization Techniques

Visualization involves creating mental images or scenarios to practice skills, solve problems, or achieve goals. This technique activates the brain's sensory and motor systems, enhancing neuroplasticity and improving performance.

Practice visualization by mentally rehearsing tasks or scenarios you want to improve. For example, if you're preparing for a presentation, visualize yourself confidently delivering the content, engaging with the audience, and handling questions with ease. Visualization can also be used to enhance athletic performance, reduce anxiety, and achieve personal goals.

### 7. Adopt a Growth Mindset

A growth mindset is the belief that abilities and intelligence can be developed through effort and learning. This mindset encourages the brain to embrace challenges, learn from mistakes, and persist in the face of obstacles, all of which promote neuroplasticity.

Cultivate a growth mindset by viewing challenges as opportunities for growth rather than threats to your self-esteem. Focus on the process of learning and improvement rather than solely on the outcome. Celebrate your progress and use setbacks as learning experiences to refine your approach and continue moving forward.

### 8. Practice Habit Stacking

Habit stacking involves linking new habits to existing ones, making it easier to establish and maintain positive behaviors that promote neuroplasticity. By associating new habits with established routines, you create a cue-action-reward loop that reinforces neural connections.

Identify an existing habit you perform consistently, such as brushing your teeth or making your morning coffee. Attach a new habit to this routine, such as practicing deep breathing exercises, reviewing a new vocabulary word, or setting an intention for the day. Over time, the new habit will become ingrained in your routine, reinforcing the neural pathways associated with it.

# Conclusion

Rewiring the brain is a powerful and transformative process that can lead to lasting improvements in cognitive function, emotional resilience, and overall mental well-being. By harnessing the principles of neuroplasticity and implementing practical strategies for brain rewiring, you can unlock your brain's full potential and achieve your personal and professional goals.

The principles of neuroplasticity are frequency and duration…in other words, consistency is the key and the more you do it the better it works.

But do not forget that working on brain connectivity should be done after the other 4 steps in the 5 step process are addressed. They do not have to be fully complete, and it can be done simultaneously, but if there are underlying inflammation, toxicity, and nutritional needs not being addressed, any progress made in brain retraining could be very short lived.  I have witnessed that first hand.

# 7

# Integrating the 5 Steps
# for Lasting Brain Health

As we conclude this journey towards optimal brain health, it is essential to understand that the five steps we've discussed throughout this book—reducing inflammation, detoxification, nourishing the body, balancing the system, and rewiring the brain—are not isolated actions but are deeply interconnected. Each step complements and enhances the others, creating a holistic approach to achieving and maintaining brain health. Addressing inflammation, detoxification, and nourishing the body often occurs simultaneously, though we prioritize reducing inflammation first to ensure the body can effectively absorb nutrients. From the first day, we can start balancing the system, and this effort can span the entire process. For some, working on rewiring the brain with brain training activities may become unnecessary after adequately addressing inflammation, toxins, and nutrition, as these foundational steps may resolve many underlying issues.

# Combining and Maintaining the 5 Steps in Daily Life

To integrate these steps into daily life effectively, consider them as parts of a continuous cycle that sustains brain health and overall well-being. Here's how to bring these steps together:

## Reduce Inflammation and Support Detoxification:

Begin by focusing on anti-inflammatory foods, such as leafy greens, fatty fish, nuts, and berries, which can simultaneously nourish the body and reduce inflammation. Incorporating detoxifying foods like cruciferous vegetables, garlic, and turmeric helps to support the liver's natural detox processes.

Stay hydrated to assist in detoxification and support metabolic functions, helping the body to flush out toxins efficiently.

Incorporate daily habits that reduce inflammation and support detoxification, such as using a sauna, practicing dry brushing, or engaging in lymphatic drainage exercises like rebounding or yoga.

It is important to engage in regular detoxification practices, such as seasonal liver cleanses that range anywhere from 3 days to a month. There are some great detox protocols out there, so if this is something you are interested in, let me know so I can help.

## Nourish the Body While Reducing Inflammation:

Specific foods and supplementation is needed in order to address inflammation and detoxification, however,  as inflammation reduces, it is important to ensure that  the body and brain receives the nutrients it needs in order to heal and thrive. This includes prioritizing foods rich in vitamins, minerals, and healthy fats that are essential for brain health, such as avocados, nuts, seeds, and omega-3-rich fish.

Supplement with necessary vitamins and minerals, especially if there are deficiencies. Minerals are highly under-utilized and need to be consumed more across the board. Methylated B vitamins (B12 and folate) are particularly important for those with impaired methylation processes, as methylation regulates detoxification and gene expression.

Consider adding natural nootropics, like Bacopa Monnieri, Ginkgo Biloba, and Lion's Mane mushroom, which can support cognitive function and protect the brain from oxidative stress and neuroinflammation.

## Balance the System Throughout the Process:

Working on bringing balance to the system can start from day one and should be a continuous effort. Techniques like stress management, regular exercise, and adequate sleep are crucial for maintaining this balance.

Integrate practices such as mindfulness, meditation, and deep breathing exercises to reduce stress and promote mental clarity, supporting both the nervous and endocrine systems. Activities that upregulate the frontal lobe (focus) help down regulate the amygdala and can bring peace and calm when experiencing anxiety and are otherwise in a state of fight or flight.

Regular exercise not only enhances physical health but also boosts brain function by improving circulation and stimulating the release of neurotrophic factors that promote neuron growth and connectivity.

Brain Gym® is a great methodology which teaches the individual how to notice their body and gives a menu of options of what to do in order to bring it into balance. If you are interested in learning about Brain Gym® please reach out.

Rewire the Brain with Cognitive Training Activities:

While some individuals may find that addressing inflammation, toxins, and nutrition sufficiently improves cognitive function, others may benefit from additional brain training activities. Activities like puzzles, learning new skills, or engaging in brain games can enhance neuroplasticity and cognitive reserve.

Focus on cognitive exercises that target specific areas of improvement, such as memory, attention, or problem-solving skills. These activities can complement other steps and further solidify gains in brain function.

There are many great technologies that specifically target brain rewiring. My favorites that can be easily done at home are Interactive Metronome® and Vital Neuro®, which can be found in the resource section of this book.

# Creating a Personalized Brain Health Plan

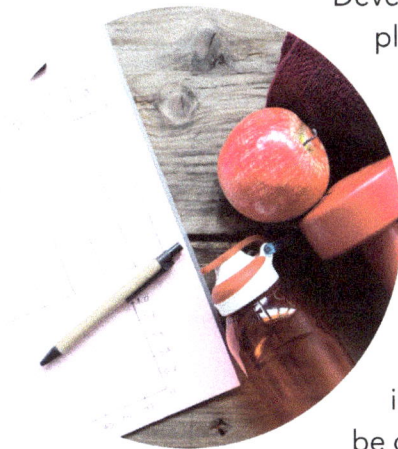

Developing a personalized brain health plan is key to achieving lasting results. This plan should be dynamic and adaptable, reflecting your specific needs and goals.

Begin by assessing your current lifestyle, health status, and areas for improvement. Set reasonable and attainable goals for yourself. It is important to remember that you will be on your health journey for the rest of your life, so give yourself some grace. You do not have to incorporate everything at once. If you try, you will most certainly fail. It is best to make a list of maybe 10 things you would like to adjust, prioritize them, then highlight the 1 thing you would like to accomplish this week. Cross it off, yet keep that one thing as part of your new lifestyle routine, and work on the next one on your list. Pretty soon you will have made some remarkable shifts.

Create a daily and weekly routine that integrates all five steps in a manageable way. Include time for meal preparation, exercise, mental activities, and relaxation. Use a journal or digital tool to track your progress and note any changes in cognitive function, mood, or overall well-being.

Be prepared to adjust your plan based on your progress and any new insights or challenges that arise. Celebrate the wins and give yourself a lot of grace.

# 8

# Additional Resources and Next Steps

It can be hard going on this journey alone. It is important to have someone that understands what your goals are, what you are trying to accomplish, and can help keep you on track. Many people find that others do not understand and may not be supportive. If this is you, you would most likely benefit from a health coach. Someone who can individualize a protocol for you and be there when you have questions or need a little extra support.

I would love to be that somebody for you!

I have everything from DIY to full all-inclusive programs.

Please visit my website, LisaAnndeGarcia.com so check out what programs I offer, or to book a call.

# Resources

Below are a list of resources of things that I mentioned in this book, and others that I think you will be interested in: *Please note that I may receive commissions on some of these items.*

1. Lifewave® phototherapy patches. These are my favorite first go-to support for anything from headache to detox. I have a YouTube video on how to use these patches to support mental health. To order patches, visit: Lifewave.com/ldegarci

2. Fullscript online supplement dispensary for discounted professional-grade supplements. You can shop here for most of what you are looking for, including products by Quicksilver Scientific (specializes in detox), and Microbiome labs (specializes in spore-based probiotics and gut restoration). https://us.fullscript.com/welcome/lde-garcia

3. Healthy Gut, for gut focused supplements that may be missing from Microbiome Labs. https://healthygut.com/LisaAnnShop

4. Cellcore, for products focusing on detox and humic and fulvic minerals. They also have a great binder for heavy metals, chemicals, and biotoxins. Cellcore.com, use code COXHC3BA in order to register an account.

5. Vibrant Blue Oils. This is my favorite Essential Oil company because of the brain based blends and other blends to support the systems of the body. "Parasympathetic" is probably her most popular blend. The store is worth checking out. https://dv216.isrefer.com/go/VBO/ldegarci

6. Interactive Metronome® is my favorite technology that helps to improve rhythm and timing, speech, cognition, and much more by connecting up different areas of the brain. This technology is not only used in schools, but in the military as well for those affected by PTSD and motor challenges. You can visit their site at

https://www.interactivemetronome.com/im-home-for-clients, but you will need a practitioner. There is an in-clinic and home version. If you would like to do this at home, please book a call so I can help set this up for you. Interactive Metronome is an option in my Comprehensive Brain Restoration package. You can find that at LisaAnndeGarcia.com/brain-restoration.

7. Vital Neuro® is an at-home neurofeedback device that is super easy to use and is very helpful in regulating executive function, focus, sleep, and helping with anxiety and other emotional issues. It can be used in as little as 5-20 minutes, is connected via an online app so that you can choose what program you would like to do that day. Vital Neuro® was designed by the creators of The Listening Program® and it uses acoustic sounds in order to adjust your brain waves. For more information, visit https://vitalneuro.com/. I would appreciate it if you reached out if you are interested as I am able to receive a small commission if I order it for you. Vital Neuro is an option in my Comprehensive Brain Restoration package. You can find that at LisaAnndeGarcia.com/brain-restoration.

# Want to go deeper?

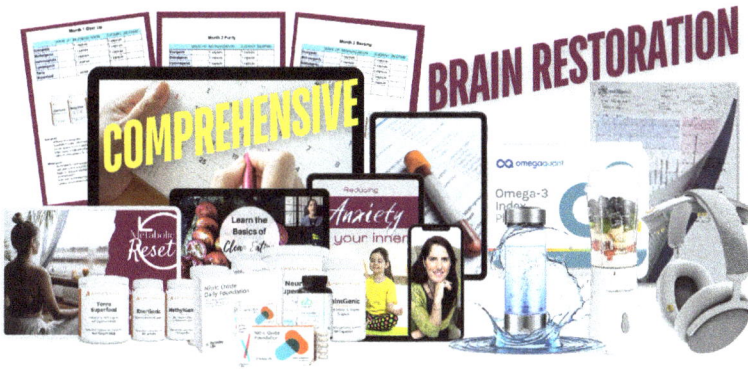

## Brain Restoration  Programs

If you have made it this far, then you or someone you love is probably struggling with one or more brain-related issues.

If you want to go all-in, then you will love one of my brain restoration programs.

- Everything shipped right to your door
- There is a size that is just right for you and your budget.
- Get email access to me for questions and support

visit the link below to learn more and enroll.

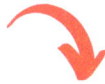

## LisaAnndeGarcia.com

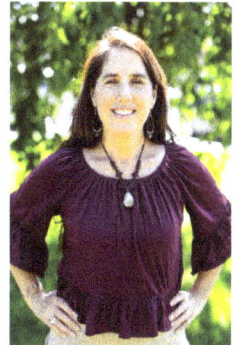

www.ingramcontent.com/pod-product-compliance
Lightning Source LLC
Chambersburg PA
CBHW062145020426

42334CB00020B/2512